EXISTENTIAL
MEDICAL
ETHICS

EXISTENTIAL MEDICAL ETHICS

RICHARD GEORGE BOUDREAU

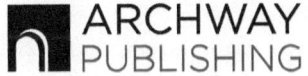

ARCHWAY
PUBLISHING

Archway Publishing books may be ordered through booksellers or by contacting:

Archway Publishing
1663 Liberty Drive
Bloomington, IN 47403
www.archwaypublishing.com
844-669-3957

ISBN: 978-1-6657-4833-9 (sc)
ISBN: 978-1-6657-4832-2 (hc)
ISBN: 978-1-6657-4834-6 (e)

Library of Congress Control Number: 2023915306

Print information available on the last page.

Archway Publishing rev. date: 9/21/2023

CONTENTS

INTRODUCTION

✖ Where Did All the Philosophy Go?

Existential philosophy has influenced perceptions of health, wellness, illness, and medicine since the ancient Greek philosophers. Multiple philosophers, from Plato to Heidegger, focused on questions about the nature of knowledge, the meaning of health, the mind–body connection, and even the influence of changing medical theories and technologies. Interpreting and evaluating these multiple theoretical foundations and the meanings they hold are important when it comes to developing, and defining, a workable philosophy of medicine.

But the problem here is that Western medicine tends to ignore philosophy, or at the very least, to downgrade it when it comes to dealing with patients. Certainly, the rapid advancements in medical technology since the 1970s are starting to lead to more reflection of the philosophy of medicine. But what's missing is the purpose of these technologies and how they can be used from a philosophical viewpoint in areas including utility and even ethics.

Let's try a simple experiment. Think about the words *medicine* and *philosophy,* then determine how these two could be interrelated. Your first thought might be that these terms simply don't match with one another. What could philosophy, and its focus on thinking and knowing, and medicine, which treats and cures people of illnesses, possibly have in common?

This question is the main problem with Western medicine today. Once upon a time, existential philosophy and medicine were inextricably linked. In the days of ancient Greece, ancient Egypt, and even during Renaissance times, the practice of medicine without some kind of philosophical underpinning simply wouldn't be considered. But as our thinking moved from the spiritual to the rational, philosophy became a focus for the humanities, while medicine fell into science. That "unlinking" we have today makes visiting the doctor because you aren't feeling very well a very trying prospect.

As a young adult, I had a family doctor who was good at what he did. He certainly knew his diseases, illnesses, and treatments. Whenever I visited this doctor for an annual checkup or illness, the situation was the same. I'd explain the situation/problem. Then he'd sit there and ponder. I often wondered if he was trying to figure out on what page of what medical text he would find the answer to my situation. While the doctor was certainly nice and an expert in his field, I came away from these appointments thinking that I wasn't a patient. I was more an object, or experiment, to which his expertise could provide a solution.

Certainly, I wanted that scientific knowledge to help me live my best life. But I also wanted that doctor to look at me as a human being rather than a medical problem to be solved. Unfortunately, this doctor wasn't unusual in his approach. Western doctors are trained to regard their patients as medical problems to be solved, rather than human beings who must live with their illnesses and diseases, and who want a solution with a little humanity on the side. This training has come about because of the dividing line between existential philosophy and medicine.

But that separation didn't just happen overnight. It required centuries of medicine's movement from the province of priests and superstitious healers to the area of reason, science, and rationality. The current age helps us live longer (though not necessarily better). The good news is that there is some movement back to philosophy and medicine.

The fact of the matter is, philosophy and medicine have

always influenced each other (Tosam 2014). Philosophy offers theoretical, methological, and analytical tools of concepts in medicine like disease, health, and care. Meanwhile, medicine provides philosophy with critical reflection issues. Part of the challenge, however, is clarifying certain concepts: philosophy, medicine, philosophy in medicine, and philosophy of medicine.

The problem occurs when Western medicine ignores philosophy and focuses just on physiology and anatomy. The problem also occurs when emotion and rhetoric trump what's best for the patient. This is what happened to Terri Schiavo.

✖ Terri Schiavo: Right to Life Versus Death with Dignity

On February 25, 1990, twenty-six-year-old Terri Schiavo suffered a heart attack in her Florida apartment and became unconscious. Her husband, Michael Schiavo, called the paramedics, but did not perform CPR on her. The paramedics did manage to resuscitate Terri, to the point that her heart was operational. Unfortunately, the lack of blood—and oxygen—to her brain had its consequences. Terri ended up with severe brain damage, resulting from heart attack-induced hypoxia. The clinical term is persistant vegetative state (PVS), and Terri remained in that state for fifteen years.

As Terri hadn't left an advanced directive, Michael, as her spouse, was appointed her formal guardian by the court on June 18, 1990. At the time, Terri's parents, Robert and Mary Schindler, didn't object to the appointment. At first, Michael's goal was to keep Terri alive, with the idea that she would eventually regain consciousness. Terri received a percutaneous endoscopic gastrostomy (PEG) tube to provide nourishment and to keep her hydrated. Several weeks following her heart attack, Terri was transferred to a skilled nursing and rehabilitation facility.

Michael attempted home care for Terri in September 1990, but she was returned to the facility after only a few weeks as Michael found himself overwhelmed. Some time later, Michael took his wife to California as part of an experimental treatment to restore her level of consciousness. This involved the insertion of a thalamic stimulator implant treatment. The procedure didn't produce the hoped-for results. Terri was returned to Florida, where she was admitted to the Mediplex Rehabiltation Center in Brandon. Throughout the early years, Terri received physical, speech, and occupational therapy, despite evidence of impaired muscle problems and difficulties in swallowing.

Over the years, the once supportive relationship between Michael and Terri's parents eroded into hostility and anger. By 1993, the Schindlers had petitioned the court to remove Michael as Terri's guardian.

Years after Terri's collapse, Michael accepted the inevitable. He realized that Terri wouldn't come out of her PVS, and that improvement was highly unlikely. In 1998, Michael petitioned the court to authorize removal of Terri's PEG tube.

This is when the familial outcry began, and spilled over into a national cause célèbre. Some might say it spilled over into an overly emotional, highly divisive circus.

On one side was Michael, who had accepted that everything that could be done for Terri had been done. His argument was that Terri wouldn't want to survive in a PVS. On the other side were the Schindlers, who sincerely believed that Terri would have wanted to be kept alive, at least until her body gave out.

The lack of an advanced directive from the PVS patient complicated matters. While the court's guardian ad litem Richard Pearse indicated that Terri had no chance of improvement, he also indicated that Terri's wishes involved "hearsay evidence from Michael," which didn't present a "clear and convincing standard" to remove the tube (Hook and Mueller, 2005, p. 1451).

The case ultimately went to trial, and for the next several years, petitions, stays, emergency motions, and appeals concerning the withdrawal of Terri's PEG flew back and forth. Terri's PEG was even withdrawn and reinserted—not once, but twice, depending on which motion, stay, or appeal was in place.

This performance played itself before a galvanized nation, with Florida being ground zero for the conflict. The Florida legislature passed emergency legislation known as "Terri's Law." Signed and supported by then-Florida Governor Jeb Bush, the legislation allowed the state to reinsert the PEG. The law was ruled unconstitutional and in violation of Michael's wishes.

Then the United States Congress intervened, forcing the Schiavo case into a federal court for review (Charatan, 2005). This is where the majority leader of the Senate, Bill Frist, himself a doctor, claimed that Terri was able to respond to visual stimuli. He never examined Terri directly, but rather, came to this remarkable diagnosis from just a few moments of a videotape that showed Terri apparently "responding" to her mother's voice and following a red balloon with her eyes.

President George W. Bush (Jeb's brother) then got into the act, noting that, while the Schiavo case underscored complex legal and societal issues, courts should come out in favor of life. While most doctors who examined Terri felt she had no chance to recover, her parents and siblings disagreed. When all was said and done on the legal side, the Terri Schiavo case involved seven years of rulings by nineteen judges and six different courts, including three appeals to the United States Supreme Court.

The case also prompted searching questions about the right to die, the right to live, and death with dignity. Also discussed was how far the state's power extended in determining whether an individual should live or die.

There was an eventual end to the emotional and legal battles. Terri Schiavo did finally die, in March 2005, fifteen years after collapsing from cardiac arrest. She died shortly after her PEG tube had been removed by the order of a Florida judge. Terri died after spending close to half her life in a vegetative state.

Close to two decades after Terri's death, we're still unpacking the meaning of it all. Her case was not the first to pit right-to-life against death-with-dignity. Karen Ann Quinlan (1970s) and Nancy Curzan (1980s) were diagnosed as being in persistant vegetative states. In Quinlan's case, her family fought for the right to remove her from the respirator. When the respirator was removed, Quinlan continued breathing on her own. In the case of Curzan, her parents fought to have the PEG removed, an appeal that was denied by the US Supreme Court but supported by a Missouri judge. The PEG was removed, and Curzan died twelve days later.

However, the Schiavo legal battle was arguably the first time that a family was split over what was best for the patient. That split played its way across the nation and involved not just the state but the nation's leaders.

As a result, Terri Schiavo's situation came down to a mix of life and politics, or what Jeffrey P. Bishop with Vanderbilt University's Center for Biomedical Ethics and Society calls "biopolitics." Biopolitics can be traced back to French historian and philospher Michel Foucault. Foucault indicated that when medicine is governed by the state, the state can wield power over life while also creating new conditions for maintenace of that life (or not, as the case might be). Terri's Law gave the state of Florida the right to keep the patient on the PEG in direct violation of the patient's husband's wishes. As the agent of the patient, it's assumed that the husband has the legal right to act if the patient doesn't have the capacity to do so.

The purpose of introducing Terri Schiavo's situation isn't to determine whether the PEG should have been removed or should have remained. It's also not to advocate for advanced directives, though if she'd had one, this might have avoided the resulting circus.

What Terri Schiavo does is bring up the idea of a "good life" versus the "bare life." Specifically, Terri had a "bare life," one that was only sustainable with the assistance of machines and nursing staff. With help from medical technology, Terri remained alive. But was it a good life? We'll delve into this later on in a quality of life discussion. But for all intents and purposes, Terri had no quality of life.

Then there's this. Let's say Terri collapsed from a heart attack in the latter part of the nineteenth century. She might have lingered for a few days, but she certainly would have died. Ventilators and PEGs weren't things in the late 1880s. Yet ironically, the late 1800s was the time when philosophy and medicine had irrevocably split—a split that would help lay the foundation of Terri Schiavo's situation a century later.

Terri's case shouldn't have generated the hysteria it did. Rather, it should have generated philosophical, thoughtful questions regarding Terri's autonomy. What, exactly, did Terri want? Unfortunately, she wasn't in a position to say, and no one truly knew Terri's wishes. But as her "agent," it was assumed that her husband likely had the best idea.

Then there was the issue involving the power of the state over an individual's life. The state of Florida was able to reinsert that PEG with the passage of Terri's Law—but was it a good idea? Along those lines, the philosophical concept of distributive justice is at play here, too. How did keeping Terri alive by artificial means impact others who might have benefitted from those means?

Then there was the issue of *personhood* and it meaning. At one time, personhood was judged by health and well-being. Quality of life meant being able to fully participate to a degree of being healthy. But these days, *personhood* could be considered a "communal attribute whose meaning is grounded in one relationship to others" (Koch, 2005). Someone in a wheelchair, for instance, might not be considered 100 percent functional. However, that individual can also interact with loved ones, travel, read a book, and be with friends. Given this construct, Terri was a person; her parents said she was. Yet to her husband, Terri wasn't a person. The personality, the soul, that made Terri a person was gone, at least from Michael's viewpoint.

This is what happens when medical technology keeps us alive without paying attention to philosophical considerations or other issues, like a body-soul connection or mind-body link. With this viewpoint, Terri Schiavo's situation shouldn't have rested on right to life versus death with dignity. Rather, it should have focused on autonomy and personhood. It should have answered questions about distributive justice and agency.

It's beyond the scope of this book to take a side in the Terri Schiavo scenario. However, what was lacking in all of the angry rhetoric and heartbreak was the philosophical, thinking side of medicine. Perhaps if calmer heads had prevailed, Schiavo might have had a more dignified end-of-life. Perhaps her husband and parents wouldn't have been on the opposite side of the legalities. In addition, maybe the issue would not have been so highly publicized—or so highly politicized.

The purpose of this treatise is to examine where we went wrong with the situation. At one time, philosophy and medicine weren't just related—they were almost the same thing. Medical treatments were conducted not just to cure illnesses but to also preserve the soul. It would have been impossible to be a medical professional without also being a philosopher. However, over the centuries, the two disciplines split and drew apart. The result is situations like Terri Schiavo's—perhaps not quite as extreme, but still there.

✄ Philosophy and Medicine: What It's All About

You've probably gathered that the challenge we face with twenty-first-century medicine is the lack of philosophy involved with diagnosis and treatment. Another issue faced is that when dicussing philosophy itself, we're taking on a hugely broad topic.

So, what is philosophy? Let's start with Britannica's (2023) basic definition. Specifically, philosophy is "love of wisdom," a "methodical consideration of reality as a whole, or of fundamental human existence and experience." All of that is quite a mouthful. It's also pretty vague. It also doesn't include the fact that there are different branches of philosophy. There's Eastern philosophy, with a focus in Budhism, Confucianism, and Daoism, to name a few. On the Western philosophy side, we have rationalism, realism, utilitarianism, idealism—and that's just a small sample.

Let's not forget religion, which also carries a philosophic bent. Basically, philosophy can be very compatible with certain religious systems; it can also involve a personal construct or a "communal understanding of proper attitude and conduct" (Mark, 2020).

From this, it's safe to say that philosophers disagree about what, exactly, they study (Tosam, 2014). To help the definition of philosophy make sense within the discussion of medicine, philosophy is described as the search for truth. It can also be defined as attempts to understand reality and to answer questions about life, knowledge, and human nature. In this sense, philosophy could be defined as a process that promotes intelligent inquiry. This is perfect when it comes to modern medicine.

Now, let's move on to the definition of medicine. It probably shouldn't come as a huge surprise that, much like philosophy, medicine has many meanings. Here's some history and etymology for you. The term *medicine* is a latin translation of the Greek term *iatrike* (Zahir, 2016). *Iatrike* is losely translated as the "art of healing." If you've heard that medicine, at times, is more of an art than a science, think back to *iatrike* and ancient Greece where this was the case.

But that's only one definition of medicine. Medicine also refers to anatomical knowledge of the human body. This isn't a "modern" definition. Rather, knowledge of anatomy as a part of medicine was introduced by Greek and Alexandrian physicians from the third century BCE and held on until well into the Renaissance period. Beginning in the seventeenth century—the age of reason—there was an increase in scientific inquiry and rationalism. While medicine supported anatomy and physiology, it entered the realms of scientific inquiry and the practice of diagnosis, treatment, and disease prevention.

These days, medicine is defined as "any substance or drug used to treat disease or injury to the body or mind."

Meanwhile, the practice of medicine involves diagnosis and treatment of a disease, disorder, or injury by any methods.

In the very early days of existential thought and healing, medical treatment and philosophy were so intertwined, it was almost impossible to separate the two. If you'd told the healers of ancient Egypt, Greece, and China that philosophy and medicine were out of synch, they probably would have laughed themselves silly.

Yet even in this day and age of science, technology, and Cartesian dualism (which will be explained later on in this paper), medicine remains an art. Medicine is an art because clinicians base their decisions on current knowledge as well as intuition and insight. As such, the art of medicine encompasses listening to and advising the patient. This, in turn, requires observation, empathy, insight, and inference. However, as we'll also see in this book, that observation, empathy, and insight tends to be lacking when it comes to the patient-physician relationship.

Part of the challenge when it comes to matching both philosphy and medicine is the requirement to clarify some of these concepts. It's also important to see how philosophy and medicine influenced one another millenia ago, when medicine, diagnosis and treatment first became a thing.

PART 1
WHERE WE WERE

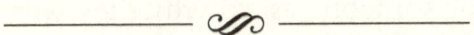

TO UNDERSTAND HOW—AND WHY—WE'RE
dealing with the issues of today's Western medicine, it's
important to understand the past—specifically, how philosophy merged with medicine in ancient times, then
split apart.

The medicine we know today has its origins thousands
of years ago, extending from from the use of plants and
herbs to heal wounds through the technological methods
of disease and other treatments today (Mantri, 2008).
Millions of years ago, our cave-dwelling ancestors likely
relied on "natural" remedies to treat sickness. If that sickness couldn't be treated, death followed. It's likely that no
one really "thought" about treatments—much of it was
based on instinct and trial and error. One plant might
kill a human being, while another might effect a cure on
issues like skin rash or stomache.

When did human instinct combine with actual, ex-testential thinking? There's no sure answer to this one, but one study noted that human-like thinking came into being around 1.8 million years ago (Putt, Wijeakumar, Franciscus, and Spencer, 2017). Fast-forwarding several million years, the simple origins of philosophy began "the first time someone asked why they were born, what their purpose was, and how they were supposed to understand their lives" (Mark, 2020). The formal ideal of philosophy is thought to have first made its appearance in Egypt around 4000 BCE with the depiction of gods and the afterlife appearing on tomb walls. By the time 2150 BCE rolled around, the philosophical treatise *The Epic of Gilgamesh* appeared.

Where does Greece come into play? After all, Greece is generally considered to be the birthplace of philosophy. In truth, existential philosophy actually popped up much earlier, during India's Vedic period (between 1500 and 600 BCE), China's Zhou Dynasty (thought to have begun around 1046 BCE), and the rise of Zoroastrianism in Persia, which was founded around the sixth century BCE It wasn't until about 585 BCE that philosophy made its appearance in Greece.

Here's another fun fact. Greece isn't the birthplace of medicine or medical treatment, though the nation does hold the origins of Western medicine. Long before Greek philosophers aired their opinions about disease, medicine, and life itself, Egyptian and Chinese civilizations had set up, and were practicing, the art of medicine.

✕ Egypt—The Launch of All Things Medical

As mentioned above, we don't know much about very early *Homo sapiens* and how they cured illnesses. However, we do know a great deal about the period of ancient Egypt, which was generally thought to be in place from 3300 to 525 BCE (Brazier, 2018). We know that "the sophisticated medical culture of Egypt...had long been known to the Greeks for its capable practitioners and drugs" (Conrad, Neve, Nutton, Porter, & Wear, 1995).

Here's another thing we know about ancient Egypt and its people: They were meticulous when it came to recording their medical observations, treatments, and medical studies (Frey, 1985). The records today are known as the papyri.

There are six papyri, spanning the period between 2000 BCE and 1500 BCE, though many of these writings have their orgins in older texts dating back as far as 3000 BCE This collection consists of the Kahun Medical Papyrus, the Ramesseum IV and Ramesseum V Papyri, the Edwin Smith Surgical Papyrus, The Ebers Medical Papyrus, and the Hearst Medical Papyrus.

These papyri tell us that the practice of medicine in ancient Egypt was highly advanced, even by the standards of Western medicine today (Metwaly, et. al, 2021). Ancient Egyptian healers had an extensive knowledge of anatomy and surgery (Metwaly, et. al, 2021). They were also highly successful in treating dental, gynecological, and gastrointestinal diseases and urinary disorders (Metwaly, et. al, 2021). These healers also knew how to set bones, treat a sore throat, handle a stomachache, and even conduct simple minor surgeries.

The philosophy comes into ancient Egyptian medicine through Imhotep.

Imhotep, Gods, and Medicine

Hippocrates is sometimes referred to the "Father of Medicine." This isn't necessarily wrong, as Hippocrates and his followers launched what ended up as the foundation of Western medicine. But Imhotep of Egypt takes the crown as medicine's "true" father (Risse, 1986).

Imhotep was chief vizier to the pharaoh Zoser, the first king of the Old Kingdom's Third Dynasty (Metwaly, et. al, 2021). He began describing the diagnosis and treatment of more than 200 diseases as early as 2600 BCE (Hajar, 2015). He became so important, and gave the Egyptian civilization so much while he lived, that the Egyptians made him their god of medicine (Sallam, 2010).

You read that correctly. Imhotep, former pharaoh vizier, was dubbed the Egyptian god of medicine. According to legend and myth, Imhotep had a direct connection to the sun god, Ra (Sallam, 2010). Furthermore, an entire cult of medicine and healing (as well as funeral rites and traditions) sprang up around Imhotep, and was eventually carried into Greek medical tradition (Risse, 1986). Imhotep was prayed to as a method of protecting against illness and death.

Here's an interesting dichotomy when it comes to Imhotep. Egyptian healers were hands-on. They had a great knowledge of healing processes, plants, and herbs. They knew a great deal about physiology and disease. They were also highly advanced when it came to diagnosing and treating disease. On top of this, Egyptian healers were staunch supporters of divine intervention when it came to health and medicine (Sallam, 2010). As such, much of ancient Egypt's therapeutic procedures didn't just involve hands-on healing, setting bones, or using herbs. These actions were backed by both religion and religious practices.

Let's take the typical ancient Egyptian patient who falls ill. From the healer's perspective, that illness was likely the result of vessels in the human body that were blocked by "foreign or noxious substances" (Metwaly, et. al, 2021). These "blockages," in turn, were the result of wounds or natural body openings. That explained the physical reasons for the problem.

The illness or disease was created by—and disseminated by—various gods, demons, and spirits (Brazier, 2018). These supernatural entities, along with the "noxious substances," were responsible for blocking the body's channels. This, in turn, prevented the body from functioning properly. The result? Illness and disease (Brazier, 2018). Neither was the impact only illness and disease. It was thought that those god- or spirit-caused blocked channels were the direct cause of mental illnesses, including dementia and depression.

On the one hand, there were the highly advanced medicines, surgeries, and other well-known hands-on treatments for all kinds of diseases or illnesses. On the other hand, prayer, worship, and a great deal of superstition were used to back medical treatments. The ancient Egyptian papyri offer multple advanced medical practices that were amazing, given the time. Each also "describes some 700 magical formulas and remedies, and contains many incantations meant to turn away disease-causing demons" (Sallam, 2010, p. 13).

As such, it shouldn't come as much of a surprise that certain Egyptian temples were created as, and used for, centers of healing. In addition to the physical methods of treating illnesses, patients (and their healers) regularly appealed to the gods. One such temple, or sanatorium, offered a series of small, dark cells, or rooms, where ill patients would be placed (David, 2008). Within these tiny spaces, patients were encouraged to enter trance-like states, so they could "approach the gods and seek healing." It might be tempting to consider these temples as the forerunner of today's hospitals, but you won't find current patients entering trance-like states as part of their healing processes.

Alexander the Great and Ptolemaic Rise

In late 332 BCE, Alexander the Great of Pella invaded Egypt, backed by an army of Macadeonians and Greeks (Samuel & Bowman, n.d.). Following his takeover of the nation, Alexander built the city that carried his name—Alexandria—in 331 BCE (Sallam, 2010). Alexandria ultimately gained a reputation for offering great knowledge thanks in part to its infamous library.

Following Alexander's death in 323 BCE, the Ptolemy dynasty ruled Egypt until the Roman invasion and the death of Cleopatra, the last Ptolemic emperor, in 30 BCE. During the Ptolemaic dynasty, Alexandria gained a reputation throughout the known world for its highly educational culture and focus on learning. The Ptolemies also saw the establishment of the Ancient Alexandria School of Medicine. Healers flocked from all parts of the known world, including Greece, to learn from this school. Many practiced in Alexandria and taught medicine there.

The Alexandria School of Medicine followed Hippocratic and Aristotelian teachings. It also successfully incorporated the advanced medical practices of ancient Egypt with healing methods from Greece. Because of its basis in Aristotelian philosophy and teachings, the institution became the first school of knowledge with philosophy as its foundation. This meant that everyone passing through the school's doors—scientists, healer/doctors, and others—were also trained as philosophers.

The main thing that Alexandria offered was reevaluation of old medical knowledge. That education also jettisoned the former superstitions that were the foundation of ancient Egyption medical treatments. Healing and medical care had their basis in logic, common sense, and Aristotlean ideas, rather than religious beliefs or even "magic."

That knowledge did not remain in Alexandria, specifically, or Egypt, in general. Many of the Alexandrian physicians coming out of this school, specifically Herophlus and Erasistratus, traveled throughout the Mediterranean basin, where they treated and taught along the way. The famous Roman physician Galen, whom we'll discuss later on in this paper, also studied in Alexandria. Galen's teachings and writings formed the basis of modern medical practices that lasted well into the Renaissance era.

To summarize all of this, the practice of medicine and healing treatments showed up in ancient Egypt, and included an emphasis on practical and natural remedies, along with prayer, ritual, and similar activities. Alexandria was established as a city of knowledge and its school of medicine offered advanced teachings. These factors moved healing from a system that was "a mixture of rational and irrational treatments, largely reliant on magico-religious procedures" (David, 2008, p. 1803) into one that focused on philsophy, logic, and common sense.

❇ Meanwhile, in China...

It's difficult to provide a discussion about medicine and philosophy without incorporating Eastern medical practices. These did have their influence on how medicine would ultimately be performed. Traditional Chinese medicine, or TCM, traced its actual rise during the Zhou Dynasty, which was in power beginning in 1046 BCE. Long before this, however, in the third century BCE, Chinese medicine was tied to three mythical emperors who were celebrated for herbal healing and other activities (Chan, Ahmed, Wang, & Chan, 1994).

One of those emperors, Huang Ti, the so-called "Yellow Emperor," is thought to have authored *Huang-ti Nei ching*, or *The Canon of Internal Medicine*, but the actual authorship of this publication isn't actually known (US National Library of Medicine, 2000). Another of the mythical emperors, Sheng Nung, is considered the Father of Chinese Medicine, and is believed to have introduced the technique of acupuncture.

From the Zhou Dynasty through the Qin Dynasty and into the Han and Tang Dynasties (ending around 900 BCE), records show an in-depth knowledge of various medical branches including obstetrics, pediatrics, dentistry, and opthalmology. There are also writings focused on setting fractures and treating trauma. Hardening of the arteries was associated with a high salt intake as early as the third century BC. Furthermore, attention to hygiene and hand-washing was in play to help avoid infection.

All of that advanced healing and diagnoses depended on a solid foundation of philosophy, and later on, religion. For example, in the first century BCE, qualifying examinations for physicians were conducted by the Chinese state. This meant that philosophy and art were incorporated into the practice of medicine, in conjunction with Confusianism, a Chinese belief system supporting personal ethics and morality.

As time went on, Daoism became an important part of Chinese medical practice. Daoism, sometimes known as "Taoism," teaches that living creatures exist in a state of harmony with the universe, as well as the energy that is found in the universe (National Geographic, 2020). This energy was known as Qi, or ch'I, and the idea behind Daoism was that individual energy and that offered by the universe were often intertwined.

This belief tied into TCM. The idea was that a healthy body was in balance. However, a body that lacked balance, for example, when someone became ill, needed a readjustment of its qi. This is where acupuncture and alchemy became useful treatments, as they restored the suffering body to balance, thereby bringing it back to the wanted state of health.

Qi supported certain medical treatments. It also held sway over diet and drugs—in other words, what was ingested in the body. Qi also stressed a lifestyle of exercise and movement, as well as calming oneself through breathing and meditation exercises (Raphals, 2020). Ge Hong, a fourth-century CE doctor, was also a Daoist who supported the use of alchemy in the area of healing. He experimented with natural drugs and even minerals to aid in the treatment of disease.

Another well-known Daoist physician was Sun Simiao, who practiced in the fifth century CE. Similar to Ge Hong before him, Sun was focused on alchemy and medicine, combining it with Daoist teachings. His writings and experiments eventually granted him the title of the "Medicine Buddha" and the "King of Medicine."

However, during the next several hundred years, TCM was gradually phased out, criticized, and ridiculed for being overly superstitious and old-fashioned. With the fall of the Chinese dynasties in 1911 and the rise of the country's nationalist government, China wanted desperately to modernize. This, in turn, led to a rejection of traditional customs, including TCM.

This was exacerbated when communism took over

China in the mid-twentieth century, and Mao Zedong continued the policies and practices that existed under the nationalist government. Under Mao, Chinese medical institutions moved away from the TCM theories and embraced Western medicine so as not to be victims of the backlash against all things traditional. However, by the late twentieth century, TCM found its way back into the more modern medical practices, though there continues to be an uneasy alliance between Eastern and Western medicine in China.

TCM is more based on balance and natural healing methods, supported by Daoism and before that, Confuciansm. The phlosophy of balance—yin and yang—was the basis of ancient Chinese medicine, and continues in the practice of that medicine today.

✕ And Finally, Greece: The Roots of Modern Medicine

When one thinks about modern medicine and its ties to ancient Greece, the automatic thought process goes to Hippocrates of Cos, who was born around 460 BCE. Long before Hippocrates came on the scene (and even before the "big three" philosophers were born), however, the the root cutters, exorcists, and others got their start as members of the cult of Asclepius, the Greek god of healing.

Asclepius, who was an actual individual before he became a cult figurehead, was first mentioned in the eighth century BCE in Homer's *Illiad* (NLM, 2012). The legend has it that Asclepius, son of Apollo, was thought to have learned about medicine from Chiron the centaur (NLM, 2012). Chiron, in turn, taught himself the art of healing when he had been wounded by Hercules.

The one reminder of Asclepius's influence on medicine is the famous caduceus of a snake entwined around a rod—these days, the medical caduceus is that of two snakes around a rod, topped off by wings. Also building Asclepius's name were various temples and shrines, all dedicated to healing; the priests were also dedicated medics, who could treat illness and disease. These temples represented the first hospital-sanctuaries, typically built in locations with the best climates and close to pure water (Bottalico, et. al, 2019). Those who visited the Asclepieion in Ancient Greece could partake of baths and massages, as well as recreational activities.

As time went on, the worship of Asclepius gave rise to a cult of traveling medics known as Asclepiads (Conrad, Neve, Nutton, Porter, & Wear, 2003). These cults traveled throughout Greece, in large and small cities and towns, in search of patients. Many of the healers also set up shop in Athens. Most healers, whether they were Asclepiads or not, obtained their medical authority not because they were qualified or educated but because they were born into families of healers. The practice of medicine was generally passed between father and son (Tsiompanou & Marketos, 2013). This meant that anyone could call himself a physician, even without training, provided he was raised within a family of doctors.

Similar to their colleagues in Ancient Egypt, Grecian healers believed that diseases were caused by some angry god or another. In other words, if someone was ill, it wasn't due to an infection or virus. Rather, it was because the gods had a beef with the patient (Bottalico, et. al, 2019).

It's also important to remember that medicine and treatment were not all superstitious rites and religious ceremonies. The Greeks studied and wrote about medicine, causal science, and disease long before Hippocrates's birth. The poet Hesiod successfully made the connection between famine, pestilence, and disease around 700 BCE. Early Greek medical authors also described diseases including tuberculosis, puerperal fever, rubella, and mumps.

Nor was there much of a dividing line between medicine and philosophy, even in the days before Hippocrates.

Alcmaeon of Croton (540–500 BC) was a well-known pre-Hippocratic physician-philospher (Huffman, 2021). In his writings, Alcmaeon supported Socrates's assertion that the brain drove the senses of sight, hearing, and smell. Socrates also had other connections with physiology and medicine.

Socrates and Asclepius at the End

Socrates, one of the "big three" Greek philosophers, was born around 469 BCE. We know much about Socrates thanks to his student Plato. It's through Plato that we understand Socrates's focus on the soul, rather than on bodies and possessions. We also know about the Socratic virtues, which are applicable to the practice of medicine today.

We also know about this philosopher's final words to his students, which called for an offering to Asclepius in an effort to give thanks to that god (Bailey, 2018). What's interesting about this is that Socrates wasn't someone who could be referred to as god-driven. Specifically, he consistently challenged the concept of gods, especially the state-approved gods that justified war, wealth, and power.

So why the plea to his students to give thanks to Asclepius? This falls directly into Socrates's belief of soul versus body. For a bit of context, Socrates was facing a death sentence in 399 BCE for denegrating the gods, and had taken the dose of hemlock brought to him by his executioner. His belief was that the body and soul are definitely intertwined, but it's the soul that pretty much drives things. As such, Socrates dubbed the soul as the "natural leader of the individual." The body, meanwhile, was little more than the container for the soul. Upon death, the soul leaves its physical prison (the body) and is successful in finding freedom and healing.

Because of this, Socrates did not fear death. Rather, he welcomed it, knowing that once he died, his soul would find the freedom it so earnestly desired. It's also perhaps why he asked his students to present an offering to Asclepius, likely in thanks for his "healing" (i.e., death). In line with the idea of healing through death, it's interesting to note that the jailor who hands Socrates the hemlock that eventually kills him is actually a pharmacist-healer. This adds to the idea that death isn't the conclusion of everything but the healing and freedom of the soul.

Another philosophical note from Socrates at the time of his death was the admonition that his followers should pay attention to their spiritual health, and make it a top priority. This is likely where the concept of "physician, heal thyself" comes from.

Plato and the Human Condition

Plato, born around 428 BCE, was one of Socrates's students. It's thanks to Plato that we know as much about Socrates as we do today. However, Plato wasn't a Socratic rubber stamp when it came to preserving his teacher's thoughts. He had his own ideas about philosophy, and especially the philosophical/medical connection.

Similar to his teacher, Plato believed that the overall focus on a human being should be on the organism as a whole rather than its parts. Unlike Socrates, he didn't view the soul as "imprisoned" by the body, with death the unlocking key. Rather, he believed that a human's physical condition was based on the connection between body and soul.

The stronger the connection, the more physically and mentally balanced a person was. Plato believed that disease or illness represented a lack of order in the body. From the standpoint of the soul, illness or disease also required more introspection. The idea here is misalignment, with the pursuit of knowledge, wisdom, and a virtuous life as the path to wellness.

It wasn't just the body-soul connecdtion that was important from Plato's viewpoint. He also noted that a patient's relationship with his or her community was also essential when considering physiological and soul-related issues (Rotaru, Popa, & Cuza, 2020). A positive relationship with friends and neighbors could support wellness, while the opposite could bring on illnesses. This isn't too different from what we know today. Studies conducted on senior citizens have shown that those who are more isolated are more likely to be prone to disease or illness.

During his lifetime, Plato wrote a great deal about medicine, medical doctrine, doctors, patients, and physicians' skills (King, 1954). Plato actually considered medicine as an art form, not in terms of the fine arts but rather as a craft in which the physician was always learning and striving to excel.

To Plato, medicine was more a model for moral philosophy rather than something involving an illness to be treated (Moes, 2001). In his works, he ties healing in with reintegration—reintegration of body and soul, and of patient and community.

Aristotle, Techne, and the Process of "Doing"

Aristotle (384–322 BCE) was first Plato's student then his colleague at the Academy of Athens. Though he was the son of a doctor, Aristotle's life focus wasn't necessarily medical-related. Howeer, Aristotle's writings on logic did support scientific and medical arguments as far ahead as the Middle Ages. Furthermore, his written discourse on psychology also attracted doctors and philosophers alike for many centuries.

Aristotle's few medical writings did expound on the relationship between medicine and health, indicating that medicine should be in place to help treat the patient, rather than the advancement of science (Bottalico, et. al, 2019). While Aristotle did share Plato's view about the unified human condition, their treatment advice differed. Plato supported the idea of balancing body and soul and body and community, with the doctor's role to help in that endeavor. Aristotle believed that physicians' skills and technical capabilities could directly help resolve some of the body-soul imbalance.

As a result, Aristotle's focus was on *techne*, a philosophical concept that refers to action, like making or doing. Techne, meanwhile, could be matched with *phronesis*, or practical wisdom. Combining both techne and phronesis, according to Aristotle, leads to a medical practitioner who is able to diagnose and treat and illness or disease. From Aristotle's point of view, the end goal of medical practice is a beneficial outcome (i.e., the patient is cured).

Given the above, it probably shouldn't come as a huge surprise that Aristotle was sometimes known as the founder and supporter of evidence-based medicine

(Sallam, 2010). It should also come as no surprise that Aristotle relied heavily on logic and the scientific method in his philosophy.

The early famous Greek philosophers supported the idea that health resulted from a body and soul that were in balance. Meanwhile, much of Greek medicine, though somewhat advanced in nature, was based on religious ritual, superstition, and keeping the gods happy (so they didn't spill their wrath on the humans).

It required Hippocrates, his followers, and the eventual Hippocratic Corpus to start medicine's move away from religious taboos to logical analysis. Even as Hippocrates moved the practice of medicine into a more logical focus, he never forgot that the mind also had an influence on how the body behaved.

❉ Hippocrates, Philosophy and Medicine

Hippocrates did not consider himself a philosopher— far from it. He's mentioned, however, for a couple of reasons. First is his undeniable influence on Western medicine. Second, while Hippocrates and his followers eschewed philosophy and any kind of religion or su- perstition in the practice of medicine, he was, in fact, a physician-philosopher in his outlook.

He's also very well known. Just about everyone, especially non-healthcare folks, know about the Hippocratic Oath. It's assumed that all doctors take, and are required to abide by, the oath before they can be unleashed on the world to practice medicine. However, just about everyone gets this wrong about the oath.

First, reciting or swearing to the oath isn't a requirement in today's American medical schools. Having said that, many of these educational institutions offer modern versions of the original oath (NLM, 2012). Second, contrary to popular belief, nowhere in the current or original oath are there the words, "First, do no harm." Finally, though attributed to Hippocrates, the oath's actual origins aren't really known; it's possible that one of his students might have written it.

Here's something else: The original Hippocratic Oath, the one taken and sworn to by Hippocrates's followers, started out with this: "I swear by Apollo the physician, and Asclepius, and Hygieia and Panacea and all the gods and goddess as my witness."

This latter fact is interesting because Hippocrates was one of the first trained healers to introduce and support natural explanations for illnesses. This was considered radical at the time, as the general consensus was that disease and illnesses were the result of spiritual or supernatural causes (Mantri, 2008). In other words, Hippocrates had little use for involving the gods when it came to medicine and healing.

So what was Hippocrates's philosophy concerning medicine? Here's what we know.

Hippocrates of Cos (460–377 BC) was born into a family of priest-doctors. He received most of his education from his father Heraclids (a physician-priest) and his grandfather Hippocrates (Tsiompanou & Marketos, 2013). I already mentioned that the practice of medicine in ancient Greece was highly unregulated, and generally "awarded" generationally within families.

While some of these doctors were skilled practitioners, just as many were "fake" physicians who fleeced customers while doing nothing to treat their diseases. This put the onus on the trained, knowledgeable doctors, who had to spend their time distinguishing themselves from the medical charlatans (Boylan, n.d.).

Enter Hippocrates who, from the start, had a different outlook on medicine, illness, and health. In addition to his refusal to connect health and divine intervention, Hippocrates spoke out against the practice of medicine as a closed occupation, only available to those few who were born into families with doctors.

In an effort to walk the talk, and to teach medicine to

the skilled rather than the related, Hippocrates established the School of Cos. The only requirements for his students were that they be willing to learn and practice the art of medicine, and that they would follow, to the letter, specific rules as outlined the Hippocratic Oath.

The ancient Hippocratic Oath (not the modified one in use used today) was a six-point statement, a contract, which required students to agree to the following (NLM, 2012).

- I will use those dietary regimens which will benefit my patients according to my greatest ability and judgement, and I will do no harm or injustice to them.
- I will not give a lethal drug to anyone if I am asked, nor will I advise such a plan; and similarly I will not give a woman a pessary to cause an abortion.
- In purity and according to divine law will I carry out my life and my art.
- I will not use the knife, even upon those suffering from stones, but I will leave this to those who are trained in this craft.
- Into whatever homes I go, I will enter them for the benefit of the sick, avoiding any voluntary act of impropriety or corruption, including the seduction of women or men, whether they are free men or slaves.

- Whatever I see or hear in the lives of my patients, whether in connection with my professional practice or not, which ought not to be spoken of outside, I will keep secret, considering all such things to be private.

The original oath has some interesting constructs that survive to this day, including dietary treatments when needed, avoidance of impropriety, and patient-physician confidentiality. There is also the mandate against assisted suicide or euthanasia, even when requested. There is anti-abortion sentiment here, as well as a touch of specialization (Hippocrates followers understood that they weren't surgeons).

The Hippocratic Corpus

From 440 and 360 BCE, Hippocrates and his students wrote a series of medical treatises which were assembled not in Greece but in Alexandria around 280 BCE (Tsiompanou & Marketos, 2013). Because of the timeline, scholars have pointed out that Hippocrates likely didn't write the entire body of this knowledge but that it was the work of several individuals.

At any rate, the fire that destroyed Alexandria's library

also destroyed many of the Hippocratic treatise; only sixty were saved from the flames. These texts were gathered, compiled, and ultimately published under the title *Corpus Hippocraticum* (*Hippocratic Corpus*). The *Hippocratic Corpus* provides an interesting window into Hippocrates's beliefs about medical treatment. For one thing, there's no doubt that the Hippocratic writers could be considered the first systematic biomedical writers in the Western tradition (Boylan, n.d.). There's also no doubt that those writings influenced development of physicians centuries later.

Hippocrates and Humors

Hippocrates was no medical philosopher or philosophic doctor. To him, *iatrike* was an already established art, which didn't require philosophy to either improve or deepen discoveries (Zahir, 2016). Despite this, his emphasis on regimen as a medical treatment considers nature, the cosmos, and the entire human form and how they interact.

The main focus for Hippocrates and his students was the four humors of the human body. The humors, consisting of blood, phlegm, black bile, and yellow bile, dictated health. Specifically, if the humors remained in alignment, a person would be considered healthy. If any of them were out of alignment, illness and disease would occur (Conti, 2012). The balance of the humors was a doctrine, one that offered healers a rational method to manage disease.

Out of the four humors, blood was considered the only one that could be controlled or manipulated. As a result, bloodletting was a regular treatment used by Hippocrates and his students. Bloodletting remained a highly therapeutic intervention to treat disease and re-store health even centuries after Hippocrates's death. In fact, in the high-tech, sterile world of today's medicine, bloodletting is useful in treating a handful of diseases.

Though blood could be released as a way to handle sickness, Hippocrates and his followers believed in diet and regimen to balance the phlegm, black bile, and yel-low bile humors. The regimen focused on all parts of a patient's life: how the patient slept, exercised, and reacted to the environment in which he or she lived. These were considered "outside influences," and were measured when dealing with patients. The emphasis on diet, especially, distingushed Greek medicine from medicine from the near east. Fast forwarding to today, lifestyle changes are also considered important when it comes to maintaining health and preventing illness or disease.

In addition to breaking the practice of medicine away

from divine actions and reactions, Hippocrates differed from his healing predecessors by relying on the signs of a patient's body to determine illness (Bottalico, et. al, 2019). To that end, Hippocrates and his students regarded illness and disease as a process, with a beginning, middle, and end. Depending on where the patient was in that process, a healer could develop an appropriate diet and/or regimen to promote healing.

Furthermore, Hippocrates supported patient-centered medicine, noting that treatment should be offered based on the patient's best interests, even if that meant non-intervention on the part of the healer. This was ancient Greece, which didn't have the life-saving medical technologies we have today, so non-intervention was probably fairly common.

However, it would be a mistake to put Hippocratic belief squarely in the realm of science and logic. He and his followers supported a holistic approach to health, combining the art of medicine with theurgical, or even religious practice based on the patient's belief system. Basically, the approach focused on not just physical and psychological care, but also social and spiritual aid. As such, the Hippocratic viewpoint considered relationships when it came to healing. These included the relationship between society and morality, between the patient and his/her spirituality, and between patient and physician.

Hippocrates and his followers worked hard to combine the practice of medicine with ethics, rational judgment, in-depth experience, and learning—not too different from the doctors and professionals of today. It would also be a mistake to assume that once Hippocrates's beliefs were immediately accepted. Certainly, he pointed out that health issues and disease were due to natural causes rather than spiritual issues. However, this approach to medicine was highly derided by Hippocrates's colleagues and peers (Mantri, 2008).

When Hippocrates came to prominence, the practice of medicine in ancient Greece was very entrenched in religion and superstition. Specifically, Hippocratic healers regularly competed with root-cutters, exorcists, midwives, bone-setters, lithotomists, gymnasts, and surgeons for patients. Hippocrates's viewpoints made it out of ancient Greece to influence medicine in the millennia that followed. Even today, Hippocrates's viewpoints concerning the whole person and the relationship between the patient and external forces are still in play today.

Hippocrates never viewed himself as philosopher, and neither did he really see how the practice of medicine benefitted from philosophy. Nevertheless, his theories concerning patient-centered management and holistic treatments are supported by the deontology school of philosophy, among others. His practice was based on ethical and rational judgment, in-depth experience, and learning.

Thought it took centuries for medicine and religion to become separate entities, Hippocrates began that split. As such, it's possible for today's doctors to trace their practice of medicine directly to Hippocrates of Cos.

✖ From Greece to Rome: Galen

Galen of Pergamum wasn't born in Greece. He was also not a contemporary of the Greek philosophers, having been born in Pergamum Mysia, Anatolia (present-day Turkey) in 129 BCE, long after the deaths of Socrates, Plato, Aristotle, and Hippocrates.

However, he is in this section involving ancient Greece and medicine because he was highly influenced by Greek philosophy and medicine. While he was born decades after Hippocrates had died, Galen followed the Hippocratic teachings, believing in a synergistic and individual relationship between each patient's body, mind, personality, and even the outside world (Mantri, 2008).

Galen's varied educational background, combined

with his outstanding education in Alexandria, among other locations, led him to insights and writings about medicine, healing, and illness, insights that lasted well into the seventeenth century. Galen's efforts, in fact, helped keep the Hippocratic focus alive, and stood as the basics of Western medicine for centuries.

Galen and Physiology

Similar to Hippocrates, Galen believed that equilibrium between the four humors was necessary for perfect health (Nutton, 2023). He took the concept even further, pointing out that each of the humors displayed two of the four primary qualities: hot, cold, wet, and dry.

He also believed that humoral imbalances could occur in specific organs rather than the entire body. As a result, he and his followers prescribed herbs and remedies to restore bodily balance by targeting specific organs.

What was unique about Galen, however, was his insistence that anatomy was the foundation of medical knowledge. Without an understanding of anatomy, it would be almost impossible to practice medicine. He agreed with Hippocrates that illness and disease had physical causes, as opposed to divine ones. Unlike Hippocrates, who believed that doctors had no business as surgeons (and had no business with dissection), Galen regularly dissected and experimented on African monkeys, pigs, sheep, and goats. He believed that dissection was necessary, both for research purposes and to improve surgical skills.

It's a good thing he proceeded in this direction. Galen's activities unearthed some never-before-considered discoveries and theories. Through his dissections, he uncovered seven pairs of cranial nerves and heart valves, and also pinpointed the main differences between veins and arteries. Galen's discoveries exploded the idea that the arteries carried air, proving that they instead carried blood.

Galen also viewed the human body as a serires of interconnected systems. There were the brain and nerves, which were responsible for sensation and thought. The heart and ateries supported energy and life. The liver and veins supported nutrition and growth.

The liver was the organ that loomed large in Galen's theories. He introduced the idea that the liver was where blood formed in the human body. From there, veins carried it to all parts of the body, where it was used as a nutrient or even transformed into flesh. In Galen's way of thinking, small amounts of blood would seep through the pulomary arteries and veins before moving through the heart.

So compelling were Galen's theories of anatomy and physiology, they carried well into the seveteenth century. They stayed in place until English physician William Harvey discovered that the heart was the seat of blood creation and circulation.

Galen and Philosophy

Another way in which Galen differed from Hippocrates is his belief in tying philosophy to the practice of medicine. Throughout his career, Galen attempted to better understand the teachings of Plato and Aristotle as a foundation for developing a perspective on the purpose of medicine. Similar to the Greek physicians, he supported the the mind/body/soul unification and its role in reaching and maintaining health.

Yet he was unique for his time in that he attempted to cure "diseases of the human soul" through physical means, generally administered by a doctor. This flew in the face of working with the soul through religious or superstitious practices. While the physical focus was important, he believed that patients should be evaluated not just through what was going on physically. Also important were issues that included emotional disequilibrium and neurosis.

The Galean Influence

Galen died in 216 BCE. As mentioned above, however, his research, discoveries, and theories formed a powerful foundation for medical practices over the next 1,400 years (Nutton, 2023).

Galen's ideas followed the spread of Christianity in the first century BCE. In fact, the Christian church appreciated Galen's theory, which was that the human body was the best design created by God. However, unlike Galen (and Hippocrates before him), Christianity also contended that disease and sin were aligned, with illness the result of humankind's fallen nature. If the soul could be cleansed of sin, then the body would follow. Despite the ties to sin and disease, early Christian physicians depended on home cures and traditional remedies in addition to prayer in an effort to heal individuals (Ferngren, 2009).

Meanwhile, the spread of Islam across nations (starting about 600 BCE) picked up on the knowledge, theories, science, and research supported by Galenic theories (West, 2014). At the same time, Arab physicians combined philosophy and spirituality with their treatments. This lasted until the end of the twelfth century, when religious dogma began to overtake logic and philosophy (Sallam, 2010).

A major benefit coming out of the Golden Age of Islam was that Galenic and other works were translated from Greek and other ancient languages into Arabic (Majeed, 2005). This helped aid the spread of medical treatments and information about illnesses and diseases.

These translations formed the basis and foundation of eventual medical learning in Europe (Al-Ghazai, 2007). The concept of the hospital was also introduced in the Islamic world, including concepts that remain today: separate wards for men and women, institutional hygiene, healthcare records, and pharmacies.

While both Islam and Christianity supported the growth of the physician, both religions also promoted the idea that physicians operated with the help of divine influence. There's little doubt that Galen's research and writings had a huge influence on the practice of medicine, both during his lifetime and in the millennia following. Galen was unique in being a proponent of physical treatment to cure disease. Through his research and experiments, he brought an understanding of how the human body functions.

Even with this focus on the physical, Galen was a physician-philosopher, through and through . During his lifetime, he sought to balance the mind/soul/body connection when it came to medical practice. He attempted to include the philosophies of Plato and Aristotle in his teachings. As such, Galen laid the groundwork for the physical medicine we know today, while he also embraced a philosophical viewpoint involving medical treatment. That philosophical viewpoint, unfortunately, is lacking in much of today's medical practice.

❈ Moving into Western Medicine: The Medicine-Science Merge

If you've made it this far, you've realized that the medicine in ancient times and the first millennia of the Common Era did a pretty good job in mixing existential philosophy and physical treatment. In fact, the viewpoint was that it would be highly difficult to separate the two topics.

Even the anti-philosophical Hippocrates believed in the idea of holistic treatment to effect cures and treatments. Hippocrates, Galen, and the doctors who followed them believed that the body and soul were an interconnected unit. Whether they subscribed to the theory that death meant the freedom of the soul (Aristotle) or that both soul and body needed attention during a lifetime (Plato), there was little doubt that the two were interlinked.

During the first thousand years of the Common Era, medicine and religion were closely tied together as well. Along with physiological advances, there were beliefs in healing miracles (Christianity) and the idea that God guided treatments by doctors (Islam).

Even through the Middle Ages and the Renaissance, as the human body was better understood, philosophy remained an important part of medical practice. In this period, Christian monks and physicians translated many of Aristotle's works from the Greek and Arabic to Latin. This supported the blending of rational medicine with Aristotalian principles in newly created European medical schools.

It was also during this time that some of Galen's theories were replaced, but not without a great deal of controversy. Belgian physician Andreas Vesalius, through the experimental method, launched anatomy as a modern science in the 1500s (West, 2014). He was, however, attacked by both the Christian Church and supporters of Galen for his viewpoints. At the same time, the theory of pulmonary transit was introduced by Michael Servetus in the sixteenth century.

While the theories and discoveries of human anatony were more in line with what's true today, the more sophisticated the knowledge beame, the more the mind-personality connection that was the basis of Hippocratic-Galenic medicine was abandoned. As early as the 1600s, physicians viewed the body as an interaction of organs. This idea found additional merit when Michael Servetus introduced the concept of pulmonary transit (West, 2014). Another seventeenth-century physician, William Harvey, made additional strides in and contributions to both anatomy and physiology.

Perhaps the greatest impact on Renaissance medicine was made by Phillippus Aureolus Theophrastus Bombastus von Hohenheim, better known as Paracelsus. Born in Switzerland in 1493, Paracelsus carries the title of Renaissance medical pioneer for several reasons. This physician-philosopher was in favor of medical observation combined with knowledge, education, and wisdom. He also introduced chemistry into the practice of medicine, though he considered himself more of an alchemist (Edwards, 2012).

He incorporated minerals into medicine, using them to treat illness and disease. It was from Paracelsus that mercury, lead, arsenic, and antinomy were incorporated into the medical arsenal. Paracelsus is also credited with inventing the tincture of opium, also known as laudanum, to help with pain.

We know today that these minerals and substances are

highly poisonous if not downright addictive. However, at the time of their introduction, they were considered miracle cures and more effective than the usual prayer or superstitous rites.

While he had the brain of the scientist, Paracelsus did lean on astrology and mysticism in treating patients. His writings were highly scientific in nature. They also included non-scientific bases so that even his preparations of chemicals sound like passages out of a grimoire.

Here's another way in which Paracelsus incorporated philosophy into medicine. He believed that the best path to perfect health was when the human and universal microcosms were in perfect harmony (Conti, 2012). In his *Opus Paramirum*, written in 1531, Paracelsus noted that this idea was based on several factors other than physiology, specifically, the spiritual, the natural, the poisonous and the planetary.

Paracelsus also went head-to-head against Galenic theories. He stated unequivocally that the four humors weren't all that important (Sigerist, 2018). In fact, many of Paracelsus's actions focused on why, exactly, people became ill. Instead of the four humors, Paracelsus believed in five spheres which determined an individual's life and health. These spheres encompassed the physical (birth and environment) and the spiritual (God and religion).

It's safe to say that, while Paracelsus was a scientist and medical pioneer, he was also deeply steeped in medicine's philosophical side, trying to figure out the spiritual and mystical sides of illnesses and disease. Though Paracelsus authored many treatises and books on medicine and medical philosophy, it wasn't until after his death in 1541 that many of these saw the light of day. Paracelsus's scientific writings were used well into the late nineteenth and early twentieth centuries, especially as they pertained to minerals and chemicals used for cures.

Paracelsus can also be thought of as representing the demarcation point between the physician-philosopher and physician-scientist (with no existential philosophy involved). He was a scientist who believed in observation and knowledge when it came to medical treatment. He was among the first to incorporate non-herbal cures into treatments. That was the "chemist" side. As an alchemist and philosopher, he believed that treatment should rely on more than just keeping an eye on the physical. He also incorporated philosophy and mysticism into his works and efforts. His spheres of health suggested that mind-body connection supported by the ancient Greek philosophers.

As such, it's safe to say that Paracelsus was one of the last physician-philosophers. During the sixteenth and seventeenth centuries, medicine was already evolving into a science and pulling away from philosophy.

The Costs of Technology and Medicine

Let's pause here and talk about the "window shade theory." The "window shade theory" relates to an historical moment of time, at least in terms of how we examine that moment in the present. Someone goes to bed one night, gets up the next morning, goes to the window, and pulls up the shade, and voila! A new era is in born. Out with the old, and in with the new. Much of the way in which we read history seems to focus on this theory—that changes in technology and other sciences were overnight sensations.

But this isn't what happened at all. There really is no such thing as a "window shade theory." This was only brought up to point out that the move from philosophy-medicine to science-medicine took decades, if not centuries. As such, someone didn't go to bed in a world in which philosopher-physicians reigned supreme only to wake up the next day to find out that these individuals suddenly dropped the philosophical side of things to become rational, logical scientists.

I mentioned earlier that Paracelsus could be considered

the dividing line between the physician–philosopher and physician–scientist. However, the overall separation of existential philosophy from medicine was much slower. That separation accelerated with William Harvey's discovery of the circulatory system in the seventeenth century.

To refresh your memory, much of physiology at the time was based on Galen's theory that blood was generated in two parts of the body. Arterial blood was created in the heart, while venous blood was created in the liver. The liver pumped blood to the entire body, while the heart only played minor role (Friedland, 2009).

Harvey, an observational scientist, didn't find that at all. In fact, he found something quite different from the Galenic point of view. In his effort to improve his research, Harvey dissected dogs and peered into their inner workings. Through this process, Harvey realized that the liver had little to do with blood distribution. Rather, the heart was the main blood-pumping mechanism. Harvey also discovered in his observations that blood flows in two loops. Instead of a flow in a single loop, Harvey uncovered the pulmonary and circulation systems.

Galen never believed that circulation was driven by divine intervention or magic, but Harvey's discovery proved it. Instead of God driving the flow of blood through the human body, physics was responsible for this movement of blood.

Harvey's efforts and research helped launch the field of modern physiology, while his efforts also supported the idea of, and need for, more experimentation in medicine. This, frankly, became a revelation to physicians. Here was irrefutable evicence that bodies operated through a mechanical interaction of organs, as opposed to some spiritual machine, or even the soul.

The rest, as they say, is history. During the next 300 years, amazing science and technological discoveries took hold around the world. Microscopy allowed an in-depth view of all kinds of things, including diseases. This understanding meant that illness and disease were no longer unknown quantities caused by some outside force. Rather, diseases were bacterial or viral, and could be treated—even cured.

Advances in surgery also allowed access to the interior of the human body. The human body became a functioning, complex organism instead of a mystery. While these important discoveries helped us understand how to fight disease and stand a better chance of survival, the process did a good job of disconnecting mind, body, and soul when it came to the practice of medicine.

This, in turn, spilled over into the training of physicians.

Medical school curricula became more focused on science, treatment, and anatomy, rather than the once humanist viewpoint that characterized how physician-philosophers operated (Doolittle, 2021). Rather than considering issues like a patient's mind, environment, lifestyle, and even connection to community, physicians were encouraged to employ their skills of observation, percussion, and palpatation, with a focus on diagnosis and prognosis.

Basically, the medical school requirements involved basic sciences and clinical training. Nowhere in the learning was there room for the humanities or phliosophy. While advances in medical technology and research have yielded some remarkable cures and methods of survival, physician-philosophers have all but disappeared.

I'll go into this a little more in the next section, but the emphasis on science versus philosophy means that physicians these days have a more active—some might say "god-like" role—in treatment.

As a result, patients seeking medical treatment are treated to objectification, commodification, and standardization (Timmermans & Almeling, 2009). This, in turn, does a good job of depersonalizing patient care. The goal isn't so much about people's needs or wants. Rather, it's about getting the job done, the diagnosis in the books, and the treatment launched.

Psychiatrist Robert Freudenthal (2021) put it best during the recent COVID-19 pandemic, especially in the early days when even the best scientists couldn't figure out how the virus was transmitted. Rather than be 'in partnership' with medical decision makers, we have become objects, he wrote, "Objects to be masked, vaccinated, tracked and traced." Those objects, he want on to say, have also become a resource for financial exploitation as well.

Accad, for one, doesn't like the change, pointing out that the last 100 years has turned the era of advanced health care into a "health care delivery system" (Accad, 2016). In this arrangement, biological materials are the inputs, with positive health outcomes the presumed output. To reach this goal, standardization and objectification became the prime modes of operation.

Does this mean we're doomed to this mechanized version of medicine? Not necessarily.

The way back to compassionate, humanistic medicine can include a greater role in medical humanities, which considers patient experience and social interaction (Have & Gordijn, 2019). Holistic health also shouldn't be mocked, but instead can be, and should be, incorporated into medical care to help promote more positive outcomes.

PART 2
WHERE WE ARE NOW

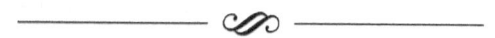

❈ We Are Machines—Apparently

THE PURPOSE OF THE PREVIOUS HISTORICAL overview was to demonstrate how medicine was once a philosophical, and even a religious and spiritual, endeavor. In addition to physical maladies, healers were careful to consider the mind and soul as well as herbs and other procedures in an atttempt to speed healing. But as scientists and physicians learned more about the human body, the idea that the mind might actually be a partner in the healing process went away. It's become easier to "fix" things that ail with scientific treatments, drugs, and even surgery. This has led to life-saving and life-enhancing technologies, but at a cost.

Here's a typical scenario. Maybe you wake up one day with a stomachache. You take the usual over-the-counter drugs to deal with it (Pepto-Bismol, anyone?). The stomachache doesn't go away, so you make an appointment with the doctor. You might be able to get in to see the doctor the same day—in most cases, it's not likely. Anyway, you go in the next day (there was a cancellation—lucky you). The doctor spends five minutes with you, asking questions and palpatating your belly. The doctor diagnoses your problem on the spot and suggests treatment. Depending on how severe your problem, that cure could be anything from a prescription antibiotic to major surgery.

Speaking of which, if the problem is something that a prescription drug might not be able to handle, your doctor will likely refer you to a specialist, who might be a gastroenterologist. That specialist will likely put you through more tests, not necessarily to pinpoint the problem, but to rule out other problems. If surgery is called for, the gastroenterologist will likely wield the scalpel. On the other hand, that specialist might refer you elsewhere, to another surgeon, for more tests, and so on. Basically, they try anything to effect a cure and make the pain go away. By this point, however, you're probably a nervous wreck, wondering how treatment of a simple stomachache could have gotten so out of hand.

Welcome to the world of Western medicine, defined as

a "system in which medical doctors and other healthcare professionals…treat symptoms and diseases using drugs, radiation, or surgery" (National Cancer Institute, n.d.).

Certainly, illnesses—and stomachaches—should be treated. It's no fun being sick or in pain. Ignore the illness and pain long enough, and real difficulties can occur. The problem, however, is that Western medicine today doesn't "heal." Rather, it attempts to "cure." But aren't these the same thing? When your stomachache goes away, doesn't it mean that you're healing?

No. There's a huge difference between "healing" and "medicine," or more appropriately, "healing" and "curing."

"Curing" goes hand-in-hand with today's medicine and medical practices. In its most basic sense, medicine is dedicated to curing, with *cure* defined as the elimination of all evidence of disease (Rankin, 2011). If your gasteroenterologist pinpoints the reason for your stomachache and treats it, you're cured, but you aren't healed.

This is because "healing" means the concept of becoming whole. While pills, prescriptions, and surgery can control disease, "most health outcomes are much more successfully treated if they are healed from the core," according to Dr. Lisa Rankin.

When it comes to your stomachache, healing involves more than prescribing pills or even surgery. These things might be involved. However, the physician who heals might also suggest dietary or lifestyle changes. That physician will also ask about your emotional state and if anything is bugging you. He or she will focus on family support. In other words, that physician looks at the whole human experience. Most gastroenterologists won't delve that deeply. It's not their fault, necessarily. It's how they were trained and molded in medical school. It's also how the current healthcare delivery system tells them to act.

Rankin also uses the example of ovarian cancer to define the difference between curing and healing. You can't wish ovarian cancer away (despite what some of the "fringe" gurus might tell you). Ovarian cancer is a disease that needs to be treated through chemotherapy and sometimes surgery. Rankin doesn't disagree that these treatments are necessary or important.

Furthermore, cancer patients aren't cured—they end up in remission, with the possibility that the cancer could recur. Rankin suggests that treating the whole patient requires addressing underlying emotional, nutritional, and life balances for a cancer patient to truly heal.

Here's the situation: While medicine is great (most times) at curing a patient, it stinks at healing. Part of it, as mentioned above, is due to training. Another reason? Your above-mentioned doctor and specialist—in fact, the entire focus of Western medicine today—operate under a concept known as Cartesian reductionism (Gold, 1985).

Cartesian Dualism: The Sum of our Parts

Sometimes known as Cartesian dualism, the concept of reductionism is as basic as it sounds. Specifically, reductionism separates the mind and body when it comes to medical treatment. Cartesian dualism supports the idea that a human being consists of two different and incompatable substances: the soul/spirit and the substantive body (Martins, 2018). These two substances are forever apart.

Cartesian dualism also considers that a body is little more than the sum of its parts. Specifically, the body isn't anything more than a machine, which is "driven by mechanical causality" (Gold 1985). In other words, similar to how an auto mechanic operates when determining why a car won't run, finding the cause and fixing it, the practice of Western medicine involves finding the problem, diagnosing it, and then "repairing" it.

If you own a car, you know a couple of things. First, cars and human bodies aren't remotely the same thing. Second, if there's a problem with your car, the chances are pretty good that the problem was caused by another problem—or that the problem is causing another problem.

For example, your mechanic might tell you that your tires are worn. The cause might be the 30,000 miles you drove on them. There could be another cause, like improper alignment, a worn-out suspension, even underinflation or overinflation. That mechanic might also tell you that your brakes need to be replaced. Yes, brakes wear out. They also tend to wear out more quickly if you regularly drive in stop-and-go traffic.

Improper alignment might cause your tires to wear out quickly. However, if the mechanic focuses only on the tires, he or she won't realize that cause. By the same token, if the mechanic doesn't ask you about how you inflate your tires (or even measure inflation), he or she won't consider that a cause either. By the same token, the mechanic might ask if you tend to "ride the brake" when you drive, which could explain why brake pads might wear out sooner than their expected life.

In this example, the mechanic looks at an entire system when diagnosing a problem. In this way, he or she not only pinpoints the problem, but can determine where that problem originated and fix that too, if necessary. If the mechanic readjusts your alignment and suggests the proper air pressure for your tires, the chances are pretty good that you won't have to have your new tires replaced as quickly.

The above is great for the full functioning of your car. Unfortunately, Western medicine doesn't take its cue from the auto repair industry. In reality, today's medicine embraces specialization, focusing on "an ethically problematic depersonalization of the patient" (Mantri, 2008, p. 179). Specifically, Cartesian dualism means that patients are viewed as just object-bodies and nothing more. The object-body concept means that medicine becomes a depersonalized experience for the patient.

"Depersonalization?" you might be thinking. "My doctor doesn't treat me impersonally. She is nice and kind. She listens to my complaints and then comes up with a solution." You're probably right. Your doctor is likely a very nice person. In the case of your stomachache, your gastroenterologist is probably also nice, as are the office staff.

The issue that your doctor and other healthcre professionals face these days is that the medicine targets your physical state only. Not much attention is paid to how you might be feeling about the pain, or discomfort, or anything else.

Let's get back to your stomachache and doctor. When you walk into your doctor's office complaining of abdominal pain, the doctor isn't going to ask you, "What is your emotional state?" or "What is going on in your living environment?" Rather, his or her main question will likely be, "Where does it hurt?" After the exam, the doctor might suggest a prescription pill or refer you to the gastroenterologist. It's likely that the pain is due to physical causes. That pain could also be the result of worry and stress, possibly caused by the fact that you lost your job the previous week.

A Side of Bacon with Descartes and Dualism

Who—or what—thought up this business of Cartesian dualism? More important, why was it even thought up in the first place?

To answer this question, let's dip back into the past again and examine the ideas of scientific thinker, mathematician, and philosopher Rene Descartes. Born in France in 1596, Descartes considered himself a mathematician first, then a natural philosopher, then a metaphysician (Hatfield, 2014).

Descartes believed that human beings are thinking individuals but that "thoughts belong to a nonspatial substance that is distinct from matter" (Hatfield, 2014). From this idea came the Latin *cogito, sum*—"I am, I exist," or as we understand it today, "I think, therefore I am" (Martins, 2018).

All of this was presented in Descartes's *Discours de La Methode*, in the section called "Methodical Doubt."

Specifically, rationalism (or rational thinking) means that no doubts exist. Implicit in this belie was that rationalism was absolutely essential in moving science forward.

Still, we need to be careful to avoid blaming Descartes alone for the advent of dualism in Western medicine, or science, for that matter. Yes, Descartes regularly distinguished the mental from the physical, but he was also a metaphysician, and all that entails. As such, he never proposed the mind/body separation, especially given his explanations that pain was definitely a body/mind issue (Duncan, 2000). What has happened is that Descartes's followers misinterpreted his writings and findings, and stated unequivocally that the successful practice of science and medicine must have a mind–body separation.

While Descartes spread his theories around France, Francis Bacon (1561–1626) was espousing his own ideas. This English philosopher was more outspoken about scientific rationalization and dualism. He was also not a fan of the famous philosophers, frequently criticizing Plato and Aristotle. Yet he also took aim at Renaissance scientists like Paracelsus (Giglioni, 2012). Bacon was a "matter man." He felt that science should focus on how matter operated; this involved use of the scientific method, along with an empirical and highly rational focus.

It should come as no surprise that Bacon's idea of

medical practice involved just a physiological focus. In fact, Bacon went on to say that physicians who didn't practice in-depth physiology when it came to curing were failed physicians (Boss, 1978).

None of this suggests that Bacon didn't care about the philosophy of knowledge and experience. He believed that any knowledge or experience should be limited solely to a specific field of application, and did not take a more holistic approach. In other words, medicine treated the physical; forget about the mind or soul.

With 20/20 hindsight, it's easy to wonder about the thought processes of Descartes, Bacon, and other scientific thinkers of the mid- to late-seventeenth century. It's easy to consider them as cold-hearted men who had little regard for the entire human experience and its importance within science or medicine.

If we consider these men in our twenty-first-century focus, we'd be absolutely right. Having Frances Bacon as a doctor would be a terrible experience. The bedside manner, alone, would probably be off-putting.

Let's, however, review these men, and their beliefs, through the lens of sixteenth- and seventeenth-century thought.

While advances were being made in science and medicine, medical treatments in the 1500s and 1600s were still largely based on superstitious beliefs and divine guidance. Spiritualism and prayer sat alongside of herbs and medical procedures. In fact, the Church still relied on healer-priests for disease and other treatments. In many cases, medical treatment and the Church were inseperable. In addition, the Church, with its focus on God and spirituality, tended to turn its nose up at scientific discoveries. These discoveries flew in the face of religion.

However, as exprerimentation and scientific discovery about the human body became more widespread, there came a split between science and religion. Medical treatments and healing were removed from the Church. It came to be that religion (and by extension, the Church) concerned itself with noncorporeal issues, like the "mind" or "intelligence" (Gendle, 2016). The body, in turn, fell under the auspices of science. As more diseases were discovered (and their causes pinpointed), cures were found to treat them, and vaccines developed to prevent them.

Accad (2016) indicates that St. Thomas Aquinas, borrowing from Aristotle's philosophy of nature, indicated that a human being represents the unity of the body and soul. In the the time of the Renaissance, however, Bacon and Rene Descartes rejected Aristotle's focus on substantial form, instead focusing on the material aspect of things.

According to Bacon, all things are measureable and quantifiable. Accad viewed the world as "nothing more than mechanical entities whose nature can be entirely understood once their material make-up is characterized." Furthermore, separating spiritual issues from the scientific side would likely help advance the practice of medicine (Gold, 1985).

It makes sense, when viewed from a contextual perspective, why thinkers of the seventeenth century favored observation and experimentation in the realm of science instead of spirituality, ritual, and religion. Removing the taboos and mysteries of medical treatment allowed science to triumph. Humans could live longer and better lives, with help from proven medicines and treatments.

This is a lovely thought. Unfortunately, the mind–body–soul separation has taken the practice of medicine to absurd extremes.

Separation: How Much is Too Much?

Here's a personal anecdote.

While waiting at an airport to take a flight that was delayed, I got into a discussion with a woman. We embarked on the usual conversation between strangers. When she learned I'd written papers about the US healthcare system, she shook her head, and told me an interesting story.

At one time, this woman's husband was hospitalized with septicemia, or blood infection. Doctors tracked the cause to an undetected urinary tract infection (UTI). A nasty side effect of septicemia is its impact on many of the body's organs. Due to the blood infection, this unfortunate man suffered a heart attack and was valiantly battling kidney failure.

Once admitted to the hospital, this man's medical team consisted of four specialists. There was a cardiologist and an infectious disease specialist, who had him hooked up intravenously to whopping doses of antibiotics. There was also a kidney doctor, or nephrologist, on hand to deal with the failing kidneys. Added to the mix was a urologist, who wanted to examine the UTI that caused the whole problem. Overseeing the team was the on-staff hospital internist, who had admitted the patient to begin with and was (sort of) keeping an eye on treatment.

What really confused the woman was her husband's need for both a kidney doctor and urologist. "I understand the need for the cardiologist and infectious disease doctor," she told me, "but the urologist and nephrologist? Don't they deal with pretty much the same thing?"

She had a point. The body's whole waste elimination system encompasses the kidneys and urethra. In today's medical world of Cartesian dualism, even these parts of the body's disposal system are cut into smaller specialties and minutely analyzed without determining how the pieces are connected. It's like calling in a plumber to deal with a clogged sink and broken faucet, only to be told that someone else would have to take responsibility for the faucet. The plumber on call specializes only in dealing with drain clogs.

If the nephrologist/urologist confusion hadn't been enough, the woman told me that things really got out of hand when the cardiologist and nephrologist ordered blood draws—for the exact same analysis. This made no sense, especially when both doctors could share their results.

That's when the woman stepped up and told all the doctors involved that enough was enough. "I told them, and the internist overseeing this whole thing, that one blood draw was necessary, especially if they were testing for similar things. My husband isn't a pin cushion." The doctors agreed (making me wonder why this whole situation had happened in the first place). The patient experienced a reduction in blood draws.

I indicated earlier that this story was anecdotal, told to me by a stranger in an airport. Unfortunately, the story is also common when it comes to the practice of medicine. Under the rules of Cartesian dualism, the body, as a machine, is the sum of its parts, even if those parts are part of an entire connected system (like the body's waste management facilities). When it comes to illness, disease, or treatment, the accepted rule is that medical specialists should be responsible only for their specific body parts.

Furthermore, it also explains why this patient experienced multiple blood tests before his wife put a stop to it. Rather than being regarded as a human being undergoing a horrific health crisis, he was regarded as a collection of symptoms: heart attack, kidney failure, and blood infection. Though the heart attack and kidney failure were linked specifically to the septicemia, the team wasn't working together from that perspective.

Here's where it gets really bad. It didn't occur to any of the specialists that multiple blood draws might be traumatic for the patient, in addition to everything else he was experiencing. The woman never said anything about it, but there's little doubt that her husband was scared out of his wits. Who wouldn't be? Picture yourself sitting in a hospital bed, at the mercy of various specialists, fearful because you've suffered a heart attack and your kidneys are on the fritz. That extra mental stress can generate certain hormones not to mention increase blood pressure (which is another problem).

There's no doubt that it took this man months to

recover physically and emotionally, but it's highly unlikely that a referral to a mental health specialist was suggested in the discharge papers. Furthermore, it's unlikely that any of the specialists, or the internist overseeing the entire situation, thought to call an on-staff psychiatrist or mental therapist on the off-chance that the patient might be experiencing trauma from the situation.

Dividing the sum of the human body by its parts, or so the thinking goes, means that each part can be taken at its own face value. Unfortunately, in the above situation—and multiple other cases—the practice of Western medicine can be considerd anagolous to the blind person and the elephant. Instead of viewing the whole of the magnificant creature, medicine tends to focus only on the trunk, back end, or tail of the animal.

We've seen what happens with this isolation, and it goes beyond multiple blood draws. Such separation fails to consider the human body as a whole when treating disease or illness. While it does understand that a blood infection can lead to kidney problems and heart attacks, it doesn't come up with a solution to help the entire situation and to make sure it doesn't happen again. It especially doesn't consider the mental, emotional, and even spiritual impacts in such a situation.

Getting back to our original premise—separating

the mind from the body—and by extension, stripping philosophy from medicine, means patients become little more than "object-bodies." In other words, doctors reduce a lively, thinking, unique individual human being into a passive entity that is little more than the sum of its parts, rather than the "centre of one's experiences, moods, expressions and thoughts." More problematically, the process dehumanizes the patient (Gold, 1985). Our patient above is more than an object of interest to several specialists. He is a human being. But he wasn't treated as such during his hospitalization.

There is a connection between mind-body separation and the absence of philosophy when it comes to treating disease or illness. Philosophy unifies mind and body and helps decision-making to that end. Without philosophy, the practice of medicine isn't all that different from repairing a car. The difference is that cars don't have souls; people do.

Healing and the Mental/Emotional Connection

The lack of a mind-body connection also dismisses the significance of an individual's mental or emotional state when it comes to physical problems or even the ability to fight a particular disease (Gendle, 2016). This isn't to suggest that an individual can wish himself or herself well if the individual is facing a cancer diagnosis. But there is a direct tie-in between an individual's emotional state and his or her physical state.

Returning to the patient with the blood infection, his physical state was dire. His heart wasn't working. His kidneys were failing. He was in pain. He was in a cold, sterile place. It wouldn't surprise me if this anxiety spiked his blood pressure while also leading to a decrease in oxygen levels. When people are nervous, they pant. Panting, the opposite of deep breathing, can curtail oxygen intake.

Let's return to another previous example concerning your stomachache and subsequent doctor visits. You're in pain, and you're understandably anxious about it. You're nervous about what might be causing the issue and might be a little apprehensive about what the doctor might find.

When the nurse takes your blood pressure you learn, to your surprise, that it's higher than normal. This is a fairly common occurrence in doctors' offices and even has a name. "White-coat anxiety" occurs when a patient's blood pressure increases while in the doctor's office. This, in turn, is caused by underlying anxieties about being outside of one's comfort zone (which a doctor's examining room is).

If white-coat anxiety can lead to higher blood pressure, it's hard to ignore the fact that there are other mental factors that impact the physical body, especially if that body is in pain. Returning to Dr. Rankin, "healing" focuses on the underpinnings of health in addition to the health itself.

As such, the nervous and respiratory systems also impact human illness (Martins, 2018). I pointed out above that someone who is anxious is panting rather than breathing deeply. This leads to a decease in oxygen. As a result, less oxygen is being received or used by the lungs. This means oxygen isn't being circulated through the body, causing a medical condition known as hypoxemia.

If that weren't bad enough, hypoxemia, in turn, can lead to other physical symptoms including the aforementioned high blood pressure. Other potential symptoms can include chest pain. Hypoxemia can also intefere with heart and brain function, while decreasing the flow of oxygen to the body's organs and tissues (Cleveland Clinic, 2023). Too little oxygen to organs can cause them to shut down; in extreme cases, hypoxemia could lead to death.

This isn't to suggest that stress or anxiety automatically bring on hypoxemia. Certainly, there are other other causes including acute respiratory distress syndrome (ARDS), pulminary embolisms, or chronic obstructive pulmonary disease (COPD). These physical issues are real.

However, anxiety over these and other medical dis-orders can generate the feeling of "airlessness," which leads to more anxiety or panic, which boosts symptoms, leading to more anxiety/panic, and so on. Trying to re-duce a patient's anxiety, which Cartesian dualism doesn't really focus on, is one step to help guide a patient toward wellness and eventual healing.

Let's take another common illness: the peptic ulcer (Johns Hopkins Medicine, 2023). Such ulcers are caused by stomach acids and digestive juices. These burn the stomach's lining, eventualy creating holes and generating pain (Johns Hopkins Medicine, 2023). The cause of these ulcers is definitely bacteria, and they are treated as such.

If you're thinking that ulcers are caused by stress, that was the once-upon-a-time belief. In recent years, research shows no direct connection between stress and uclers. Notice I said "direct." No, there's no causal relationship, but research also proves that stress can weaken a body and its immune system. There is such a thing as "stress colds." When a body is stressed, it's less able to fight the viruses, including cold viruses, that are constantly circulating around us. As such, stress also inihibits a body's abiliity to heal from bacteria, including the ulcer-causing kind.

The treatment for a peptic ulcer is medicinal. That's the "cure" part. A really savvy gastroenterologist might also recommend lifestyle changes to the patient to ensure that the stomach heals and the bacteria causing the problems become inert. These changes might include eliminating smoking and adding more fruits and vegetables to the diet. That doctor might also suggest that the patient increase physical activity and practice meditation or mindfulness. The "curing" part of peptic ulcer treatment involves the drugs. Meanwhile, the patient "heals" by making those lifestyle changes, and especially by taking steps to reduce stress.

The problem here is that Cartesian dualism bases its activity on biological reductionism of disease. This, in turn, supports medical practices that aren't successful in supporting either wellness or healing (Gendle, 2016). They might "cure" an illness or disease, but they do not ensure that the illness or disease won't return. Ongoing diseases and illnesses might generate profits, but they don't do anything to help an already overstressed healthcare system or help a patient's well-being and overall health.

Understanding—and Treating—Pain

Pain is especially counfounding to Western medicine and its focus on Cartesian dualism. Sometimes pain can be tracked to a physical cause, and that cause can be dealt with. Other times, there might be absolutely no physical reason for pain.

How is pain defined?

In the late 1970s, the International Association for the Study of Pain defined pain as "an unpleasant sensory and emotional experience associated with actual or potential tissue damage, or described in the term of such damage" (Arnaudo, 2017, p. 1083). But the definition also pointed out that "pain is subjective." In other words, pain can take place with a definite cause. It can also occur without any obvious reason.

Here's one thing we do know. Pain is a physical phenomenom. A doctor's typical response to a patient who presents with pain symptoms is to prescribe a painkiller. In the stomachache example above, the "cure" was either a prescription or a referral to a specialist, who would then "treat" the symptom.

Over-the-counter painkillers are fine for muscles strains or backaches. Stronger pain medicine, like hydrocodone or Tylenol with codeine, are effective for surgery-created pain.

However, there are times when the pain might not come from a specific, physical cause, but this is about as far as Western medicine will go with it. An "outside-the-box cause" of pain occurs only when that symptom and its reason doesn't fit into a doctor's range of specific knowledge. In this situation, the doctor concludes that the pain is all in the patient's mind.

If you've been paying attention up until now, you might be perking up and saying, "Yes! The doctor is acknowledging a likely mind-body connection to pain! Now the doctor can look for other options to treat this poor patient's suffering."

Unfortunately, Western medicine doesn't treat a patient with a "mind-related" pain very well. According to the doctor's knowledge, the patient is probably imagining the pain. This means the doctor might refer said patient to another specialist—a psychiatrist, psychotherapist, or psychologist. There is no effort on the part of the doctor to determine why or how the mind or emotion might lead to a physical manifestation of pain. There is no effort to believe the patient, who is experiencing the very real sensation of pain. Instead, the patient is told that he or she is crazy (or at least, it's implied that there's some mental disconnect) and that the doctor can do nothing.

For that patient who is in pain, there's nothing worse than the implication that the hurting is all in the patient's mind. Even worse is the implication that the patient is dreaming up symptoms as a way to get attention. The patient who is in pain knows something is wrong. The patient can't function because, well, pain. Yet Western medicine's path is first to determine a specific and pin-pointable cause. Second, if there is no obvious cause (i.e., no tissue damage or anything else apparent), it must be psychological. In the latter case, let the mental health experts "cure" that psychological issue, and the pain will go away.

More often than not, psychological treatment doesn't do squat. It only convinces the patient that he or she is alone in the battle, and the medical establishment couldn't care less about what is really wrong.

This can especially be the case with chronic pain, which is defined as "pain that lasts longer than the usual course of an acute injury or disease" (Arnaudo, 2017, p. 1086). The problem here is that the pathological issues involving chronic pain aren't 100 percent understood, again, because there isn't any obvious cause or reason for it.

This relates to the philosophical field of anti-realism, which is something that will be discussed late on in this paper. In cases like fibromyalgia, volvodynia, and Lyme disease, there is no apparent or physical reason why some-one should be in pain. At one time (and even today, among some doctors). these health issues were lumped in the category of "mental."

Let's examine fibromyalgia. This is defined as "a long-lasting disorder that causes pain and tenderness throughout the body, as well as fatigue and trouble sleeping" (NIH, 2023). Fibromyalgia also generates an increased sensitivity to pain. The symptoms can range from sleep problems to headaches (including migraines) to anxiety to overall pain and stiffness. Furthermore, these symptoms can manifest differently in each individual.

The problem, however, is that there is no direct cause or reason for the pain and exhaustion that fibromyalgia generates. That lack of specific, scientific evidence makes it more difficult to put fibromyalgia in a neat and tidy "diagnosis" box.

Some research does show that fibromyalgia is linked to a central nervous system disorder or even possibly a rheumatic condition. Furthermore, imaging studies have identified various altered signalling in neural pathways in fibromyalgic patients (NIH, 2023). There's also some indication that this disease has a genetic foundation; if a parent suffers from it, it could manifest itself in the child.

Additionally, fibromyalgia is often tied to a co-morbid mental state like depression. Furthermore, fibromyalgia can occur in tandem with lupus, rheumatoid arthritis, and even chronic back pain or irritable bowel syndrome.

However, its varied symptoms and causes are what

make fibromyalgia so difficult to diagnose and treat. This is frustrating for both patient and doctor. For the doctor, an inability to get a handle on a specific cause of pain—no apparent injury! no diseased tissues!—means that trying to actually cure the problem is practically impossible. Let's remember that Western medicine is in the business of "curing" patients rather than "healing" them. The only explanation for the various symptoms (at least from the doctor's point of view) is that the cause is psychological.

For the patient, this lack of causation is especially frustrating, not to mention heartbreaking. The patient is already struggling with chronic pain, fatigue, and any number of other symptoms. However, because the doctor can't pinpoint the cause of the pain, it apparently doesn't exist. The patient is informed that there really isn't anything wrong, and maybe the next step is to talk to a mental health professional. The pain, which is very real to the patient, is in in her head. Not only is she in chronic discomfort, she must now prove to the medical establishment—and herself—that she is sane, and that the pain she's experiencing isn't all in her head.

Yes, I said, "she." Fibromyalgia, along with chronic fatigue syndrome (CFS) and other similar disorders, tend to affect women more than men. Gender bias is a regular topic in healthcare, because women are believed to be more emotional and more "sensitive" to symptoms. CFS, fibromyalgia, and other similar diseases appeared in the twentieth century. Yet many doctors, espeically male doctors, treated them like the "hysteria" of the nineteenth century—as a "female" condition, with no physical causes. In the eyes of the medical establishment, the pain is linked to "female issues."

In short, pain needs to have a physical reason for its existence for it to actually be diagnised and treated. Without that reason, "it's likely to be treated with scepticism and moral approval, or be attributed to a psychiatric condition" (Duncan, 2000, p. 508).

How else should non-organic pain be treated? It could be focused on as a holistic issue. This isn't to suggest that someone suffering symptoms from fibromyalgia will be "cured" through holistic healing. A doctor with a holistic viewpoint can take the time to understand the patient's experience with pain and its impact on daily activities. Symptoms can be treated with medication and alternative therapies like massage or even acupunture. The doctor might also suggest certain lifestyle changes in diet and exercise.

Meditation and mindfulness could also be recommended. Rather than dismissing the pain due to lack of cause, a doctor considering a holistic method understands that a patient is indeed suffering, and then works on ways to help mitigate the pain.

Again, this won't lead to a cure. It does, however, assure the patient that she's not being treated like someone from the tin-foil hat brigade. If she has specific steps to take to help alleviate or mitigate that pain, this could help her overall emotional viewpoint as well. This is the antethesis of Cartesian dualism, with a focus on the holistic and on healing.

The Rise—and Practice—of Evidence-Based Medicine

Another way in which Western medicine continues to move away from a mind-body-soul connection is through a concept known as Evidence-Based Medicine, or EBM. The idea behind EBM is that the best scientific and medical evidence should be relied on when diagnosing and treating patients (Masic, Miokovic, & Muhamedagic, 2008). The term was coined in the early 1980s by David Sackett and his team of epidemiologists at McMaster University in Canada. They sought to advise physicians and clinicians about how to best use and research medical literature (Thoma & Felmont, 2015).

The implication behind EBM is that because the evidence has been proven again and again through research and clinical trials, it will work with populations that present with similar medical problems. Because it works with one group of people (or different groups of people), it will work with everyone.

There is some good in the EBM philosophy. For example, if a patient presents with a high cholesterol level, the EBM suggests that diet, exercise, and medication can be the keys to lowering "bad" cholesterol levels.

Then there are the patients who present with higher levels of "bad" cholesterol, and nothing provided through Western medicine works. Cholesterol medication, diet, exercise—none of these work. How could this be? EBM says it should work, so what's going on?

What's going on is that not all patients are alike. Some might just be stuck with high cholesterol. It could be that the baseline for certain patients is higher. EBM doesn't necessarily support any of this.

One main criticism of EBM is its overreliance on what's been done in the past, and then the tendency to put those solutions in stone with the assumption that they will work for an entire patient population. That assumption is false. There will be the outliers who can't be "cured" from EBM research. Sometimes the so-called "causal" mechanism promoted by previous evidence just won't work.

This is not to suggest that EBM isn't a basis for diagnosis and treatment. Western medicine can go too far with it, however, and assume that because "evidence" is available for treatment, it will work for anyone walking into a doctor's office and presenting with specific symptoms. EBM is a good tool—but it isn't the only tool that can, or should, be used.

Healthcare Delivery— The Guaranteed Body-Object

Then there's another problem with medicine, and that's the issue of how the service is delivered. When you went to your doctor with the stomachache, you were likely allotted about fifteen minutes to spend with the doctor (and the end result was that you probably had less than five). This slot of time gives the doctor just about enough time to go over your symptoms, examine you, suggest treatment, and then move on. It doesn't give much time to explore other factors that might be the causal agent of your stomach pain.

Healthcare today is delivered through assembly-line methods, with diagnoses "coded" for insurance reimbursement purposes. While assembly lines are great for manufacturing processes, they are not all that great when it comes to treating humans who are sick or ailing.

Let's return to the early days of Western medicine in the United States, around the late nineteenth and early twentieth centuries. At that time, doctors did have offices and office hours, but they also made house calls. There were good reasons for this. In a predominantly agrarian society, people couldn't take the half-day necessary to hook the horse up to the cart and ride into town to see the doctor. Even as the industrial revolution and mechanization took hold in the cities, house calls were the accepted way of treating patients, well into the 1950s.

The benefit of housecalls is that they gave doctors bird's-eye views into their patients' lives. These family practitioners could take in a patient's personal environment and observe family interactions. If the farmstead had three or four kids running around with runny noses and the patient was suffering from the same thing, the doctor had a clear diagnosis—and he could tell everyone to isolate in an effort to prevent further contagion.

Another benefit from this delivery style was that the doctor, more often than not, would treat multiple generations of the same family. In some cases, that doctor even delivered many of the babies. In this case, familiarity didn't breed contempt. Rather, it bred knowledge. The doctor understood the family's lifestyles, work schedules, interactions, and home life. They could make informed diagnoses on a holistic basis. The patients, in turn, trusted the doctor. After all, if the doctor had treated Grandpa, delivered a mother's baby, set a father's broken leg, and helped deal with an infant's croup, who could be more trustworthy when it came to diagnosing and treating various other ailments?

There are many reasons why the house call went out of fashion. One prevelant theory is that the doctor's time became too valuable to waste in making house calls. They simply weren't efficient. The costs of traveling and waiting were transferred to the patient. Specialization is also suggested as a reason for dwinding house calls.

It goes without saying that it's the extremely rare doctor who makes house calls any more. It's important to point out that house calls weren't a wonderful panacea of health care. There were downsides. The doctor could only bring a limited amount of equipment to a housebound patient. Furthermore, there was the issue of resource distribution. A doctor who spent the night at a patient's bedside wasn't available for other patients.

The point here is that house calls helped the doctor develop a strong relationship with patients and an understanding of their environment. Today's office-centered care does not. These days, patients don't have many interactions with their doctors. Some more conscientious patients might have an annual physical. They'll visit the doctor if they're ill or are hurting, but generally a patient won't visit a doctor more than a few times a year.

Additionally, today's healthcare system and delivery methods are predicated on cost-effetiveness, public and private healthcare insurance systems, and limited financial resources (Chrousos, Mammas, & Spandidos, 2019). Furthermore, the healthcare system is in the hands of private insurance, which is responsible for patient coverage and doctor remembursements.

Because of this, doctors have a limited amount of time to spend with patients. They just don't have the time to spend a half an hour with a patient and find out that maybe the inidividual is experiencing a high level of stress at work, or that a child is being bullied at school—that is, unless the patient actually volunteers this information. Many times, patients don't, because it might not occur to them that there's a connection between what they're experiencing physically and some totally unrelated, but underlying, cause.

This isn't to suggest there's no room for the medical

tools we enjoy today. It's great to know that no one needs to suffer the ravages of polio, or that cataract surgery can provide a patient with new vision. Scientific knowledge is necessary to succeed in the practice of medicine.

Furthermore, use of EBM can combine with that science knowledge to build a foundation for a patient's diagnosis. The operative word here is "foundation." Science and EBM should be the start in patient treatment. The doctor should build on that foundation with what he or she might know about the patient, rather than simply taking the scientific, or Evidence-Based Medicine, viewpoint.

A Better Focus—The Lived Body

We know a lot about migraine headaches. From a scientific perspective, we know that migraines are the result of brain activity that temporarily impacts the nerve signals and blood vessels. We also know that sometimes people will experience great pain with their migraines, and require a darkened room and plenty of quiet until the pain goes away. Other times, they might experience something called an "occular migraine," when vision goes fuzzy for a brief period of time but no pain occurs.

What causes the brain to react in such a way? Surprise—there is no one specific cause when it comes to migraines. For one patient, stress might be a trigger. For another, a gift box of dark chocolates creates the problem. Aged cheeses, red wine, exhaustion—there are many things that can trigger migraines. Just handing the patient a bottle of pills and telling him or her to lie in a dark room might treat symptoms. However, without in-depth knowledge of a patient's behavior or lifestyle, it doesn't get to the root of the problem. It doesn't focus on ways to help ensure that the migraine doesn't occur in the first place.

Yet this is how Western medicine works. It treats humans as "object-bodies," mechanisms that are totally separate from human experience and intelligence. From the object-body viewpoint, migraines cause pain, and that pain should be treated with a pain pill.

Here's the problem with the object-body focus: First, it relies on the idea of Evidence-Based Medicine and "proof of pain" when it comes to diagnosing and treating illnesses and (Mantri, 2008). Rather than exploring other reasons when it comes to determining the reason for the medical issue, the idea here is physiology or bust. If nothing appears to be wrong, then there is nothing wrong.

This leads us to the second problem: the voice of the patient is silenced. The patient knows he or she is not feeling well. It's up to the doctor to pronounce whether something is wrong or not. This takes away a patient's power over his or her body, and even over his or her feelings. Instead, the doctor is thought to know best. And the patient? Well, the patient is just an object who doesn't have the medical knowledge or skill of a talented doctor. It's little wonder that the current state of Western medicine is thoroughly frustrating to a patient, something I'll explore in greater detail later on.

What's the solution? One thought is that Western medicine might be better served by regarding the human body as a "lived-body." The object-body separates experience and intelligence from the physical. But the lived-body concept examines everything about the human: the mental, physical, and emotional aspects.

The doctor who follows a lived-body concept for a migraine-plagued patient will ask about the pain. That doctor will also ask about the patient's lifestyle, and what he or she was doing before the migraine came on. Other questions might include what's worked in the past to relieve the discomfort. This is a patient-doctor dialogue, rather than a doctor pronouncement. At the end of it, the doctor might still prescribe the pain pills, but he or she might also suggest that the patient lay off the red wine for a couple of weeks, or practice mindfulness to relieve stress or tension. Based on the results, the patient could incorporate those functions into his or her particular lifestyle.

From the above example, it's possible to see that the "lived body" takes in everything about the patient: physical, emotional, and, to an extent, spiritual. The lived-body concept also considers the quality of the doctor-patient therapeutic alliance.

The lived body state is what doctors and patients should strive for. As has been made clear, Western medicine tends to be uncertain about "the role of the psyche" when it comes to treatment. Disease doesn't—and shouldn't—exist independently of a patient's life and world (Tosam, 2014). Someone can be ill without actually having a specific biological cause. Psychosocial factors can also account for disease (Tosam, 2014).

In short, modern medicine has concentrated on the disease to the exclusion of all else, especially the patient. Today's doctors treat disease and patient as two separate entities. A doctor who focuses on the lived-body concept, on the other hand, can better understand what exactly is going on and the best way to treat an illness. The patient isn't "cured" of a medical malady, but that individual can heal and find the way to health.

✷ What Happens Without Philosophy?

Health and the "Health Care System"

Let's explore the idea that Western medicine today tends to leave the patient out of the whole realm of diagnosis and treatment. Rather than trusting that the patient knows what he or she is talking about when discussing symptoms, the assumption is that this isn't the case. It's the doctor who knows it all. The patient is just a sideline. This definitely discounts the idea of a body-mind-soul connection, too.

The earlier example of the hospitalized man with septicemia illustrates the "patient-knows-nothing-doctor -knows-all" philosophy. From the doctors' points of view, the man wasn't a living, suffering patient who suffered from an infection and horrific organ failures. Rather, he was someone to be poked and prodded, nothing more than a body offering information like blood pressure, respiration—and blood, itself. This continued until the wife stepped in to remind all concerned that the man was a human being, not a pin cushion.

Here's another example, a case study presented by Zapata and Moriat (2015).

A patient, Mr. F., was admitted to a New York City

hospital with a significant, hacking cough. The patient
had a history of coronary artery disease and had already
experienced a mycardial infarction, or heart attack.

Mr F.'s admitting physician was Dr. C. She planned
to discharge this patient as soon as he demonstrated that
he was comfortable breathing without assistance. On the
Friday morning of Mr. F.'s planned discharge, Dr. C. received a call from the patient's cardiologist. It seemed as
though Mr. F. was scheduled for a repeat stress test and
echocardioagram. This wouldn't be a problem for most
patients. However, the heart doctor explained that Mr. F.
lived alone in Brooklyn. He had no access to transporta-
tion, so getting him back to the New York City hospital
would be very difficult.

The cardiologist feared that these factors meant that
Mr. F. wouldn't return to the hospital for the much-
needed tests, which were scheduled for the following
Monday. Would it be possible for Dr. C. to keep him in
the hospital over the weekend, to ensure that the patient
would be present for the Monday tests?

Dr. C. told the cardiologist she'd think about it. She
did. She ultimately charged him. First, some of her sal-
ary, and her overall advancement up the hospital hiear-
chy, meant keeping patients' hospital stays to a minimum
number of days. Dr. C. wasn't thinking totally of herself

when deciding to discharge Mr. F. If Mr. F. were to remain in the hospital over the weekend, he could be at risk of hospital-related infections. In his current shape, such an infection could cause severe problems for the patient.

Finally, there was the question of resources. Specifically, given that the tests conducted by the cardiologist were on an outpatient basis, keeping Mr. F. in the hospital meant fewer resources would be available to other patients who might have a greater need for an inpatient bed.

In describing this screnario, Zapata and Moriates pointed out that Dr. C's situation isn't unique. This decision-making process is something that healthcare providers face on a daily basis, and most times, more than once a day. There's been enough in the news about hospital-related infections, like methicillin-resitant Staphylococcus aureus (MRSA), to raise concerns over the safety of hospital patients. As such, keeping a patient hospitalized simply to ensure he would be able to have his tests done when they were scheduled could generate more problems and concerns, not just for the patient, but for the healthcare system charged with treating him.

Was discharging the patient actually the best outcome for all concerned? For Dr. C., probably so. But for Mr. F., not so much. He would now have to find a way to get to the hospital as an outpatient. It was specified that his ability to do so wasn't all that certain. Because of that difficulty, it's possible that Mr. F. wouldn't have bothered with the tests. That, in turn, might have led to more heart issues, another inpatient hospital stay, and reduced quality of life (or death).

It's certain that Dr. C. went over all of these outcomes in making the keep-or-discharge decision. What's interesting to note in this case study is that Mr. F. wasn't asked or consulted about this situation. There's no proof that the patient was approached and asked what his preference would be.

It could be that Mr. F. might have jumped at the chance of not having to stress about returning to the hospital on Monday for his tests. He would be right there, and there wouldn't be worry about bothering a neighbor to drive him, or coming up with the money to take a cab back into Manhattan. Conversely, he might have decided he was tired of hospital food. He might have been missing his home and familiar surroundings. He might have already lined up a ride back into the city on Monday.

We have no way of knowing, because apparently Dr. C. didn't think to ask Mr. F. what his preference might be. It didn't matter. All that mattered was keeping the hospital stay to a minimum.

Though the above is a case study, discharging patients

early these days isn't unusual. In fact, the goal of hospitalization is to free up beds as quickly as possible. This
is fine, if the patient is truly feeling better and is ready
to go home. In most cases, patients don't want to stay in
hospitals longer than absolutely necessary.

As was the case with Mr. F., patients don't get a choice.
They can check themselves out early, but then they have
a large red "AMA" (against medical advice) on their re-
cord, mainly to protect the doctors from any liability or
lawsuits. On the other side of the coin, patients are often
discharged from hospitals long before they're ready.

This was especially the case with the so-called "managed care" revolution of the 1990s and early 2000s, which
saw the rise of health maintenance organizations (HMOs).
The goal was to prioritize cost-cutting measures. Yet the
managed care movement received a backlash from both
patients and physicians. Patients, objected because HMOs
limited what service providers they could see and rein-
forced the perception that faceless corporations were in
charge of their treatments (Mechanic, 2001).

Meanwhile, physicians claimed that the "assembly
line" nature of their practice (only allotting a certain
number of minutes to each patient, no matter the sever-
ity of the illness or disease) was eroding their ability to
provide correct treatment (Mechanic, 2001). Then there

were the sensationalist media stories, which portrayed still-sick patients who were discharged early from hospitals, and women who were discharged on the same day on which they'd given birth.

Regardless of whether these issues were true or not (Mechanic, for one, claims much of this was blown out of proportion), managed care was forced to reform. But some thirty years after the end of the managed care experiment, doctors still can't view the patient as a partner in his or her own treatment and/or health. Even more interesting, patients are becoming better advocates for themselves, thanks to the internet.

There are times during which that "doctor-as-all-knowing-individual" can be a problem. Getting back to the case study above, Mr. F. could have advocated for his own position. He could have suggested to Dr. C. that he remain in the hospital to ensure he'd be tested. It's still possible that Dr. C. would have opted to discharge him, but maybe the patient and the doctor could have worked out a solution to the problem of getting him back to the hospital for his tests. Through this process, Mr. F. could have some semblance of control over his own health issues.

From a philosophical viewpoint, Zapata and Moriates noted that

Shared decision making can be an important strategy for ensuring ethical and high-value care decisions when there is not one clearly superior treatment option, since achieving greater alignment of care with patients' values has the potential to improve patient understanding and satisfaction, result in better outcomes, and reduce unwarranted variation in care and costs. (1024).

The problem, the authors pointed out, was that prioritizing the patient's preference might conflict with other issues, like limited health resources (i.e., a hospital bed) that someone else might need. There's no easy solution to this, but the point is that doctors need to be forthcoming with their patients and involve them in the decision-making process regarding their health.

Defining Health, Medicine, and Healthcare

Speaking of health, here's another issue. *Health, healthcare,* and *medicine* are frequently interchanged and interrelated. But how, exactly, is *health* defined?

Take a moment to think about this. If you come up with a blank, you're not alone, so let's turn to the dictionary. The basic definition, as offered by Dictionary. com (2023) is that health can be described as "the field concerned with the maintenance or restoration of the health of the body or mind." However, this doesn't tell us what *health* is.

Here's what the World Health Organization (WHO) has to say about health (2022).

> Health is a state of complete physical, mental and social well-being and not merely the absence of disease or infirmity. The enjoyment of the highest attainable standard of health is one of the fundamental rights of every human being without distinction of race, religion, political belief, economic or social condition.

Perhaps unsurprisingly, the WHO's definition has come under fire for being too vague. Under this definition, someone with a chronic disease could be considered unhealthy (Bradley, Goetz, & Viswanathan, 2018). Let's put it this way: one person's "highest attainable standard of health" is not another person's. Someone suffering from a terminal illness might have a "highest attainable standard of health" for that particular condition, but still need to take pills to survive. Furthermore, under this definition, if *health* is defined only as the absence of disease, it stands to reason that only a doctor can determine if an individual is healthy (Sartorius, 2006).

Stephen Hawking, arguably one of the twentieth century's most brilliant minds, was diagnosed with motor neurone disease in his early twenties. This disease results in an extremely short lifespan, measured in months. Yet Hawking outwitted the medical prognosis, dying when he was seventy-six years old. Confined to a wheelchair, unable to really talk or even care for himself, he would have been considered "unhealthy" by the above standards. Yet he functioned extremely well in his environment and worked around his limitations to become a famed expert in his field.

Let's broaden the concept of health and define it as:

- The absence of disease or impairment;
- A state that allows an individual to cope with daily life demands; and
- A state of equilibrium an individual establishes within himself and his social and physical environment. (Sartorius 2006, page number)

Let's also keep in mind that not all three points above are necessary for good health. Someone could be restricted to a wheelchair and still be perfectly able to cope with daily life demands, and establish equilibrium in himself or herself and within the social and physical environment. This brings us back to Stephen Hawking.

While the definition presented by Satorius is more in line with what health should be, part of the problem we face today in Western medicine that *health* is strongly connected to the concept of *healthcare*.

Now I'll ask again: what is healthcare? Again, if you come up with a blank, don't feel bad. Googling the term *healthcare* generates millions of hits and (it seems) just as many definitions. The American Medical Association Code of Ethics (2003) tells us that basic healthcare is "a fundamental human good" that enables "our opportunity to pursue life goals, reduces our pain and suffering, helps prevent premature loss of life, and provides information needed to plan for our lives."

This is fairly clear, but what it lacks is how that "fundamental human good" should be delivered, or how it should be handled.

Now, going that final step, what is medicine? As mentioned earlier, *medicine* also has a broad definition. Here, we'll point out that medicine is actually a subset of healthcare. While medicine focuses mostly on treatments and methods to "cure" physical ills and disease, healthcare deals with everything else. Healthcare focuses on handling disease, along with considering a patient's well-being.

The problem, however, is that what we know as healthcare is actually medicine. The patient with septecemia didn't benefit from healthcare. His well-being wasn't considered. Nor was Mr. F.'s well-being taken into account in the above case study.

Yet despite all of this, health is connected to healthcare. This has led to a system in which patients are catagorized according to their diseases and financial status (Bradley, Goetz, & Viswanathan, 2018). Instead of being viewed as thinking, feeling individuals who need assistance in achieving their best version of "health," today's patients are viewed as little more than cost generators.

Under this model, people are viewed as expenses rather than assets This version of healthcare focuses on disease treatment and sick care, rather than prevention and wellness. It also means that philosophy is stripped out of the practices of healthcare. Even worse, a physician who is unsuccessful in this model—in other words, that doctor can't "conquer" a particular disease—is considered a failure, both individually and as part of the system in which he or she operates.

A better definition of health needs to step outside of

disease and how medicine tries to fix things. Health is less about any kind of disease and more about being present in the moment, feeling fully alive, and in an optimal state of being based on current conditions.

The Lack of Philosophy—and its Downsides

How, exactly, does philosophy fit into all of this? How, exactly, does the study of knowledge, reality, and existence pair with the practice of medicine?

The simple answer is that it should. The study of knowledge and understanding of reality should go hand-in-hand with disease and illness treatment. It's probably easier to answer this question by explaining what philosophy doesn't do when it comes to the practice of medicine (note we don't say "healthcare" here).

Philosophy does not:

- Narrow a patient to a body-object or a machine that is solely the sum of its parts;
- Focus on only physiology or cause-and-effect; or
- Forget that the individual behind the illness or disease is a flesh-and-blood individual who has likes, dislikes, fears, and other emotional aspects.

The practice of medicine without some kind of philosophical component is a highly impersonal process. Its mandate involves specialization and the "doctor-is-all-knowing" attitude without the understanding that the patient can be a valuable partner in determining his or her health issues.

Without philosophy as a foundation, current medical thought assumes that nature is governed by both the law of physics and by linear causality. Linear causality is the belief that "if this happens, then that occurs." In other words, a treatable disease or illness is one that has an obvious cause. Because of the medical industry's focus on nature, physics, and causality, the human body is "defined as matter, subject to natural law and as such, completely explorable by means of fragmenting methods" (Kirkengen, et al., 2016, p. 497).

Here's a very recent example of how, exactly, this happens.

During the dark days of the COVID-19 pandemic, the if/then causality was made highly apparent with this ultra-contagious disease. From a basic standpoint, unvaccinated people stood a higher chance of getting COVID and dying from it. Therefore, if an individual was to be vaccinated, there would be less chance of contracting the virus.

But here's another if/then from the COVID-19 annals. If people are isolated for too long, then their mental health will suffer. Let's put it this way: During the shelter-in-place/stay-at-home lockdowns, some people used the time to better themselves. They exercised, lost weight, started and finished crafts, and enjoyed family time. Others, however, did not. Cut off from their social circles, these individuals ate too much, didn't exercise, and become more and more depressed. Even when some of the lockdown restrictions were lifted, these individuals couldn't pull themselves out of isolation. Many remained depressed and despondent.

Added to this were the millions who were "vaccine-hestitant," who refused to wear their masks in public, and otherwise eschewed the "science" that was said to limit contagion. This isn't to suggest that this population cohort was correct in its assessment. It is a stark reminder that the "medical" minds failed to consider the overall well-being of this population. Medicine (specifically, scientific medicine) couldn't conceive that anyone would be stubborn enough to refuse vaccines to prevent illness or masks to prevent the spread. It labeled this crowd as "stubborn," "opinionated," and even "stupid," simply because it failed to listen to reason. Scientific medicine also dubbed this cohort as selfish; after all, if

EXISTENTIAL MEDICAL ETHICS   97

they would receive the vaccine (and wear masks), it meant the disease wouldn't spread to other people.

In truth, vaccine-hesitant people weren't any more stubborn, opinionated, selfish (or even stupid) than those who willingly found a vaccine center and happily rolled up their arms for the jab. They had different viewpoints and concerns about the vaccine and potential side effects. From this perspective, a better way to deal with the vaccine-hesitant population would have been to regard them as human beings with their own opinions and viewpoints, rather than as a group of stubborn, spoiled toddlers who thought of no one except themselves.

How vaccine-hesitant people were handled during the pandemic lends truth to the idea that in today's world of medicine, the person has been "systematically eliminated in accordance with the scientific tradition, which is still dominant" (Kirkengen, et al., 2016, p. 498). Furthermore, the pandemic proves that Western medicine embraces "a materialistic and mechanistic ideology that reduces the patient to complex body machinery" (Have & Gordijn, 2019, p. 165).

The primary focus is only on treatment and cure, which ignores the life story and wider context in which a particular illness or condition might exist. Adding to this issue is a lack of time for interpersonal communication and care fragmentation. The result is patients who feel dehumanized.

Let's get back to the COVID vaccine-hesitant. With this medicine mentality, it's no wonder they fought back against the jab. Many were hesitant because the mRNA vaccines available hadn't undergone the usual years of experimentation and tests. They weren't sure what the side effects might be. Rather than providing information that might assuage some of these fears, doctors dismissed the concerns. This led to an information gap, which was filled by misinformation, gleaned through social media and other non-official sources. The rest of the story is stark and awful—the unvaccinated who were infected by COVID were more likely to die.

Trusting the Doctor—or Not

COVID-19 presents an extreme example of how today's medicine works holistically. Here's a more common one. You have a patient with physical problems, who approaches the healthcare system in hopes of getting help. Instead, she feels as though she's little more than a mechanical curiosity to a doctor. The doctor takes note of symptoms and pronounces a cure in less than five minutes—that is, if there's an obvious cause. If the problem is more complex, she'll refer the patient to another doctor, a specialist. In this scenario, things are more depersonalized. The patient isn't a whole person. She's a foot, or a knee, or a back. The patient is little more than a part to be treated and cured.

If there is absolutely no proof of any cause for the patient's complaints, the next stop might be a mental health professional. Here, the patient is informed that whatever is ailing her is likely an emotional issue rather than a physical one.

With either path, the patient isn't in power. Rather, she's at the mercy of a doctor who has control over her symptoms. That loss of control can lead the patient to believe she doesn't matter. She feels like just another case—one of many. If referred to a physician specialist, the patient will likey undergo a battery of tests to rule out what might be wrong. Even this process is highly impersonal (sitting still for an hour while undergoing an MRI isn't one of life's greatest thrills). A diagnosis and treatment might be rendered, based on Evidence-Based Medicine, without a thought for non-physical issue that might impact a patient's ability to be compliant when it comes to treatment.

Even worse, if there's no obvious cause, and the referral is to a mental specialist, the patient might start *doubting herself and her own symptoms. Maybe this is all in my mind,* she might think. *Maybe I am—crazy.* The resulting frustration, anxiety, and depression become a self-fulfiling prophecy.

In either case, this dehumanization process erodes a patient's trust in the doctor. After all, how can an individual confide concerns or fears in someone who doesn't show much empathy or interest, whose only thought is to find the cause of an illness and to treat it? Patients often find they have to prove that they aren't feeling well, and that physicians don't believe these patients' complaints (Au, Capotescu, Eyal & Finestone, 2022).

Another issue is that depersonalization and dehumanization can lead to a higher degree of medical error (Haque & Waytz, 2012). There are instances in which the medical process of today can result in pulling up the wrong patient file—or even performing surgery on the wrong body part.

None of this does anything to make the patient feel better about being treated. In fact, the opposite is true. If a patient who goes into the hospital for knee replacement surgery has to worry that there is a chance the surgeon might operate on the incorrect knee, this only adds to the stress and uncertainty of an already stressful and uncertain procedure.

Practitioners, Burnout, and Depression

It isn't only the patient who suffers from the de-personalization of Western medicine or a the lack of a mind-body-soul connection. Though it might not seem like it on the surface, doctors and nurses also suffer from the mechanized focus of today's medicine.

Let's get back to the discussion about medical errors and patient mix-ups. This is definitely problematic for patients. It's also emotionally draining for doctors and nurses. The consequences of a mistake or error can be catastrophic. There is a high degree of self-blame in this situation for such a failure. There are also lawsuits, which can be costly and in some cases, could end a career.

Plus there are often "post-mortems" that uncover more serious medical errors (especially those resulting in a patient's death). Though these "morbidity and mortality" conferences are meant to focus on what caused the outcomes and are meant not to punish, doctors are human. When discussing the causes of errors, self-blame can still rear its ugly head.

The current system also erodes the faith of many physicians in their power to do good for patients. In most cases, individuals go into medicine in hopes of two things: to make money and to help others. Many picture themselves as offering empathetic and compassionate care.

The process to be in a position to provide that care, however, takes years. Medical school itself requires a four-year commitment. Then there are internships and residencies, which can extend the timing by up to an additional seven years. Within this period of time, students and residents are subject to intense education and trial-by-fire training, complete with relatively low wages and a general lack of sleep (especially during residencies).

By the time they become full-fledged MDs, these individuals are fully trained scientists. However, their empathy and compassion have been squeezed out by multiple sleepless nights, contempt from older, more experienced staff, and general uncertainties about whether they might be fit for the job. In an effort to hide these uncertainties, many doctors become arrogant and unsympathetic. To them, MD can mean "major deity."

Furthermore, health care delivery doesn't permit enough time to connect with a patient outside of a physical complaint or two. Ironically enough, those doctors who take the time to do so receive complaints from patients who say they had to wait around for an hour to be seen.

As a doctor, you're darned if you do, and you're darned if you don't. If you don't take enough time with patients, you're considered unfeeling and remote. If you do spend more time than the allotted fifteen minutes with a patient, you likely hear from other patients who are waiting, and an office staff that needs to keep things moving. It's little wonder that doctors in this system become detached from the people they're paid to diagnose and treat. They become indifferent and numb to concerns or suffering. They also suffer from feelings of dehumanization. They're not doctors; they're simply "medical professionals."

Unlike the practice of medicine in the days of Hippocrates, medicine today is science and "take a number." It's no longer an art. For the doctors who entered the field with the desire to help and heal, this rude awakening has led to burnout, depression, and frustration, all of which takes its toll on patient care. In extreme cases, the assembly-line-like nature of our healthcare system has caused some doctors to commit suicide.

Equitable Justice and Healthcare?

A lack of philisophical existentialism involves more than doctors and patients. It also impacts public health and population groups.

In theory, the practice of medicine is supposed to embody justice in addition to respect for patient autonomy, beneficience, and nonmaleficence, concepts we'll dicuss later on. However, justice isn't really served in the current healthcare system. Healthcare is supposed to embody "fiscal sustainability of the health system for the greater good of society" (Zapata & Moriates, 2015). In reality, the current US healthcare system is far from sustainable. There are vast populations that don't have access to quality healthcare, due to expense and lack of resources.

For those who do have the means and the doctors, the healthcare system isn't much easier. Patients who are ill, especially those who are chronically ill, find themselves navigating both medical systems and social structures that weren't developed and aren't maintained with their best interests in mind.

As mentioned frequently throughout this paper, the biomedical focus is on the "object-body" as opposed to the "lived-body." Also inherent in this experience is a term known as "medical gaslighting." Medical gaslighting is supported by "largely unchallenged ideologies underpinning healthcare services" (Sebring, 2021, p. 1951). Unfortunately, medical gaslighting also means that the doctor, who is medicine's spokesperson, has the right to determine what's real (diseases that have an obvious cause) and what isn't (disorders or diseases that seem to have no cause). Basically, the patient presents symptoms.

The doctor determines whether those symptoms are legitimate and "deserving of recognition by the medical system" (Au, Capotescu, Eyal & Finestone, 2022).

For patients to be treated, they need to have cultural health capital. Specifically, they need to know how to report their symptoms to be taken seriously, and to access the healthcare they need (Collyer, Willis & Lewis, 2017). It goes without saying that not all patients have that cultural health capital, which means that patients who have problems or symptoms might not be able to access the care that they require. This is in the hands of the doctor "gatekeeper," an individual who has the power to determine if the patient is truly ill or not.

Another problem here is that patients end up in a system that requires multiple tests designed to rule out potential diagnoses. Each ruling out leads to more uncertainty about the patients' conditions, putting patients in positions of uneasiness. From a philosophical point of view, the process tends to downgrade patients' moral statuses, especially in terms of epistemic injustice (Blease, Carel & Geraghty, 2017). Specifically, because knowledge is withheld from the patient due to any cause or because treatments are uncertain, this leads to a form of injustice to the patients.

Far from being a system that combines patient care

with fiscal responsibliity, the US healthcare system is costly and inefficient. Additionally it demeans the patients and generates burnout among the doctors.

❦ Then There's Quality of Life

For many people, "quality of life" is a black-and-white issue. It pushes a lot of buttons. You either have a life you live to the fullest or you don't. Next time you're at a party or are meeting friends for lunch, ask around. Ask the partygoers or friends if they would be willing to live in a vegetative state. The chances are pretty good that most of those you ask would say absolutely not. If their lives aren't ones in which they're aware, then their loved ones should just go ahead and pull the plug.

Asking your friends about mere survival versus actual life is anecdotal, but there's research to back it up. Polls and surveys repeatedly point out that people don't want to live if they're in a vegetative state or otherwise not able to consciously participate in life (Kitzinger & Kitzinger, 2012). Furthermore, families of those who are severely brain-injured have indicated that keeping them alive through artificial means is "a fate worse than death."

Why did the Terri Schiavo case generate such controversy and divisiveness? Why would anyone want to keep alive a woman who so clearly was not living her best life? Even more important, why would anyone want to keep Terri attached to machines for survival, when she'd already told her husband that she never wanted to be kept alive in the situation in which she ended up?

First, Schiavo's parents were convinced that the doctors were wrong. They had doubts that their daughter really was in a minimally vegetative state. They knew that Terri was "in there" somewhere, and it was only a matter of time until she regained full consciousness and would pull out of her coma, or whatever it was.

The right-to-live supporters agreed. Those who supported the idea that Schiavo would ultimately come out of her situation saw short clips of her apparently "interacting" with others (Breed & Crenson, 2006). Those clips also showed Schiavo potentially "reacting" to her mother's voice and visually following the bouncing of a red ballon. These were the clips that made it on the evening news. They're also the clips on which Senator Bill Frist (himself a doctor) made his claim that Terri was indeed "alive."

But here's the issue: patients in persistent vegetative states do show reaction to stimuli. This is the body reacting, without any conscious thought involved with it. Even patients who are brain dead continue to respond to stimuli. The thing is, they have no conscious awareness of doing so. The response is a physiological action. There's no "there" there in people who are brain dead. Many times that's the case with PVS patients, as well.

Michael Schiavo finally faced the facts, acknowledging that his wife simply wasn't aware of what was going on. Terri wasn't there anymore. Jay Wolfson, one of Schiavo's many guardians during the heated court battles also noted that (2006), "Ms Schiavo was as old as she was going to get when she died. Her husband and many others, argue that she 'left this world' the night of her collapse in 1990."

Wolfson's conclusions come from the autopsy of Schiavo's brain after she died. He pointed out that the "degree of atrophy and damage to her brain was profound," even worse than some had thought (Wolfson, 2006, p. 4). There was no evidence of trauma that caused the brain damage.

The question I ask here is whether Schiavo's quality of life justified the means to keep her alive, as well as the ongoing court battles and the removal and reinsertion of her tube. Again, this happened twice before the final removal. It's not the purpose of this paper to position an "either-or." Rather, it's to address quality of life and health and how they fit into the existential philosophy realm.

Schiavo's situation was extreme. She was in a persistent vegetative state. Because of the conflict between family members, decisions about what to do with her entered the legal and political realms. The overall issue was less about what made sense for Teri, and instead focused on right to life versus death with dignity. The philosophical issues of autonomy, beneficence, nonmaleficence, and justice didn't seem to enter into the equation.

In the time of Hippocrates, a Terri Schiavo issue simply wouldn't have existed. From the time of ancient Greece until the early part of the twentieth century, a person with a brain injury or other major injury wasn't kept alive by artificial means; the technology wasn't available to do so. These days, there's talk of a "window of opportunity" in conjunction with brain injuries or even brain death (Kitzinger & Kitzinger, 2013). That "window" is actually described as a period of time when withdrawing or withholding any kind of medical intervention can allow a patient to die. This terminology is used only in extreme cases, for patients whose survival prolongs dying instead of patients who might be restored to a semblance of acceptable life.

In this case, "quality of life" is pretty straightforward. A patient with an unrecoverable brain injury, or brain death, doesn't really have much quality of life. The decisions are rarely so black and white. Let's take the bed-bound person with severe dementia who has no family or friends and is confined to a board-and-care facility. This individual might be viewed as having a life of poor quality. She can't get up and walk. No one comes to see her. She's locked in her brain. It could be said that being locked in her brain, she might have happy memories, and so a positive quality of life. In this case, the body is still being treated. The problem is that the mind and soul aren't necessarily living their best lives.

As such, quality of life is important when it comes to issues like health care delivery, medical treatment, and even distributive justice. Unfortunately, quality of life in medicine is a hugely complex issue.

An Understanding of Quality of Life (QOL)

These days, quality of life ranks up there in importance with medical diagnosis and treatment. In fact, it's considered an important target in the fields of health and medicine (Haraldstad, et al., 2019). Understanding QOL is essential when it comes to improving symptom relief and providing care and rehabilitation of patients. QOL is also useful for anticipating future problems for patients.

Here's a brief history of the concept. The term QOL

was first mentioned by J.R. Elkington in 1966. At the time, he noted that medical technologies (like transplantation) raised questions about how a clinician should protect a patient's quality of life (Elkington, 1966). There was also a touch of philosophy in Elkington's queries. Specifically, these queries focused on what resources should be put into which programs to achieve the most in health and quality for the highest number of individuals in society.

During the 1970s, physicians used QOL to decide on health issues, like relying on aggressive treatments to extend life (Pennacchini, Bertolaso, Elvira, & DeMarinis, 2011). The questions asked involved what sacrifices might be involved when increasing longevity. This moved into some treatments' side effects and whether those effects were worth it to prolong life.

By the 1980s, QOL was used to guide decisions about whether to limit treatments in an effort to better allocate healthcare resources. In the years following, as the number of treatments expanded, more specific and systematic evaluations were necessary when it came to efficiency and effectiveness. This was due to increasing expense of healthcare. As such, attempts were made to consider broader definitions of health status, rather than recovery or survival, when it came to treatments.

Today we continue to ask ourselves about the definition of QOL and how it fits into healthcare and treatment. How can we define it so it makes sense?

The World Health Organization defines it as "an individual's perception of their position in the in the life in the context of the culture in which they live and in relation to their goals, expectations, standards and concerns" (WHOQOL Group, 1995).

Reducing this to a simpler definition, quality of life can be defined as how well an individual is able to enjoy normal life activities (Stoppler, 2021). On the medical front, "some medical treatments can seriously impair quality of life without providing appreciable benefit, whereas others greatly enhance quality of life."

Delving further into the topic, there is also health-related quality of life (HRQOL). This is defined as the impact that disease or disability has on functioning. In other words, HRQOL determines if a person's health status can support his or her ability to live a good and fulfilled life (Haraldstad, et al., 2019). Again, as pointed out earlier, "health" is a highly subjective term. One person's disability might be considered "not healthy," but the individual is still getting the most out of life despite his or her limitations.

Then there is the other side. I had a diabetic patient

who had his legs amputated. Though this required some adjustment, he eventually was able to function well. He had a loving wife, wonderful children, and a job he enjoyed. He was content.

Then, as can happen with diabetics, his heart and kidneys began to fail. He began dialysis treatments for his kidneys. Then the doctors suggested open-heart surgery. This man and his family then had a decision to make. Because of his amputation, he used his arms for maneuverability, but the heart surgery would have rendered his arms useless. As the procedure involves wiring the sternum, patients are told not to use their arms or to raise them high for weeks afterward. This meant the patient would be bedbound for weeks, possibly months.

Because of this, he decided against the surgery. He didn't want to put his family through the lengthy recovery period or have them remember him as a bedbound, helpless invalid. He told me he'd rather spend the time remaining enjoying his family and dogs rather than face being bedbound and continuing to deal with end-stage renal failure and diabetes. He died six weeks later. Certainly, the open-heart surgery would have prolonged his life, but he wasn't happy with the quality of life that might have resulted.

Someone else with the same issues might have decided on a different path. That individual might have felt that "where there's life, there's hope." Certainly, the process would mean immobility and ongoing kidney and diabetes treatments, but at least (the thinking might go) he or she would be alive. The person would still have brain function and the ability to talk with his or her family. To this individual, quality of life would be much different than it it was to my patient.

Though QOL is well-meaning, it's hard to measure, especially when dealing with medicine and treatments. Certainly, there are instruments that specifically target a "good" life versus a life of struggle. However, because QOL, and especially HRQOL, are such personal issues, these measurements can only help so much.

A well-known example from the literature involves cancer of the larynx. In most cases, patients with this disease are raced into either a laryngectomy or radiotherapy as treatments. Laryngectomy offers the best chances for survival, but it also means the cancer patient won't be able to talk any more. Radiotherapy doesn't have this problem, but the chances for survival with this treatment are much lower. Research by McNeill and his colleagues has shown that some people for that reason prefer radiotherapy, while others have less problems with adjusting to alternative forms of speech (e.g., oesophageal speech) and prefer laryngectomy (McNeill et al, 1981). QOL, in this case, is a personal preference.

The Philosophy of QOL

It should probably come as no surprise that various philosophers have attempted to address QOL with medicine. Consequentialism states that an outcome determines the viability of an action. As the name suggests, the focus is on the consequences of an action, rather than the action itself (Sinnott-Armstrong, 2019).

An action, like a doctor treating a patient, has a consequence. The patient (hopefully) gets better. In applying consequentialism to my diabetic friend, he understood that his action (electing not to have the heart surgery) would lead to a specific outcome (his almost immediate death). That was preferable to another outcome (the likelihood he would be bedbound for a long period of time) if he'd taken the action to have heart surgery. He understood the consequences of both actions.

My patient understood the limitations of his life. Consequentialism becomes more difficult in other situations. For example, during the 1980s, consequentialists addressed the issue of babies who were born with very severe handicaps. These babies weren't expected to survive long, and they appeared to be in great pain. Among the consequentalists, this situation justified infanticide. The thought here was that keeping these poor babies alive served no purpose other than to prolong the infants' pain and the parents' anguish.

There is another side to this thought. Many believe that souls are born into this life for a reason, even if that reason is suffering and pain. They would have disagreed with the consequentalists that survival was not an option for these babies. The babies were born for a purpose, the argument went. Their very existence, no matter how painful or filled with anguish, was the purpose.

This is where religion and spirituality can also impact the quality of life focus. I mentioned earlier that religion and medicine were hand-in-hand centuries ago, and that suffering was an important part of illness. That idea carries over today. Some religious or spiritual beliefs do underscore suffering as an essential path to a glorious afterlife. In other words, many religious faiths support withdrawal of treatment and/or life support among patients who are brain dead or who have terminal illnesses (Chakraborty, et., al, 2017). Others frown on doing so. This is the "quality of life" versus "life-at-all-costs" argument. It's also the argument that puts suffering, or a poor quality of life, against death with dignity, or a life free from pain.

The philosophical viewpoints of hedonism and welfarism are also tied to the QOL debate. Many tie hedonism to other issues, like overabuse of food or substances, or extreme materialism. The actual philosophical idea behind hedonism is that humans are motivated by pleasure or pain. While pleasure has worth or value, pain doesn't have any value—it's the opposite of worth (Moore, 2013). My patient mentioned above was more motivated by the pleasure of spending his last weeks on earth with his family. The pain of open-heart surgery was not one he wanted to contemplate.

This could fit in with the beliefs of 1980s hedonist philosopher Helga Kuhse. Kuhse was dead set against the idea of "sanctity of life," or life at all costs. In her discussions, she focused on the moral difference between intentionally discontinuing ordinary medical treatment and intentionally discountinuing extraordinary medical treatment.

She and Peter Singer, also a hedonist philosopher, pointed out that survival, no matter what, was a false viewpoint. They argued against the idea that all human lives, no matter the quality or kind, must be considered valuable and should not be violated. According to these philosophers, there should be a definite link between the patient's quality of life and his or her best interests (Kuhse & Singer, 1989). A poor quality of life wasn't in anyone's best interest, they said. In many cases, they believed, euthanasia would be in the person's best interest.

QOL and the Euthanasia Decision

During the late twentieth century, Jack Kervorkian made headlines for championing terminal patients' right to die through physician-assisted suicide. Kervorkian, a pathologist, assisted more than 100 patients to their ends, losing his license to practice medicine and being charged with murder in the process. These days, eleven states in the United States provide medical aid in dying, but each state has its own legislation when it comes to such medical aid.

By the same token, there are those who believe that this process is a cop-out. In discussing euthanasia in the face of possible poor quality of life, cardiologist Richard Fenigsen (2011) believes that one person's quality of life can't be compared to another's. In writing about euthanasia to end suffering, he explains that suffering is relative, adding that "doctors and all people of good will should seek to relieve suffering, not exterminate the sufferers" (p. 247).

His belief is that to present a seriously ill patient with the idea of an "easy death" allows that patient to view his or her suffering as unbearable. "People," he writes, "have an admirable ability to reconcile themselves to suffering" (Fenigsen, 2011, p. 246). According to Fenigsen, there are stroke victims who can enjoy all the small pleasures of daily life "and beam with happiness when visited by a grandchild." There are also those patients with intestinal cancer who empty their own colostomy bags on a daily basis and have happy marriages and regular activities.

He is absolutely correct in that one person's QOL is not another's. He also offers good points about loved ones perhaps trying too hard to coerce terminally ill relatives into euthanasia to avoid the burden of care. He also blames society for making suffering a terrible thing. Most people, he points out, suffer, but get on with life.

Here's the problem with Fenigsen's argument, however. Not all stroke patients have "little pleasures" or even grandchildren. Not all patients with intestinal cancer have happy marriages or even want to be part of an existence in which they're constantly having to empty their fecal bags. Let's get back to the woman who was mentioned earlier, the woman with Alzheimer's who is bedbound and who doesn't have friends, family, or even a home. Is this someone who is able to reconcile herself to the pleasures of daily life? Is this someone who has regular activities other than eating and diaper changes, as if she were an infant?

How should QOL be measured in this woman's situation?

This is where welfarism comes into play. The basic belief of welfarism is that nothing matters more than the well-being of individuals (Keller, 2009). Welfarist philosophers tend to link happiness with life. But "happiness" is also difficult to measure.

Let's put it this way: Alzheimer's is an awful disease. This form of dementia robs an individual of important memories. The patient who has Alzheimer's can forget loved ones, and can even become hostile or angry with those around him or her. The question here is how can someone with this disease be happy or content? What is the welfare of this individual?

To the family and loved ones of the Alzheimer's patient, the disease might seem to be terrible and a fate worse than death. The patient, however, might not actually be suffering, especially if he or she is well cared for. The patient doesn't know that he or she has forgotten anything. The patient is likely living some pretty good memories, which keeps him or her content.

But the Alzheimer's/demetia debate opens another

philosophical issue, that of autonomy. Leaving an indivdiual in the advanced stages of Alzheimer's by himself or herself can be dangerous. Yet once you introduce a caregiver into the situation, or put the patient into a memory care cener, you're eroding that person's autonomy in the name of keeping him or her safe.

Measuring QOL

This gets us back to the question of how, exactly, quality of life can be measured. Early measurements focused on how "normalyl" a patient functioned after treatment (Nantais & Kuczewksi, 2004). This model became more important as medicine became more concerned with clinical protocols, costs, and resources. Additionally, standardized models exist to supposedly examine QOL objectively. One such model is the quality-adjusted life years, or QALY. These are ranked on a scale from 0 to 1. 0 means death, while a score of 1 signifies a year of healthy life.

Many times, decisions to treat a patient (or not) depend on how much such treatment might improve a patient's score on the QALY scale. However, while QALY might determine a patient's physical state, it might not fuly represent that patient's actual quality of life. There are factors other than health that are weighed when it comes to QOL.

Then there's another solution: ask the patient. Doing this requires regarding the patient as a partner in his or her medical treatment. It also includes a patient's autonomy emphasis (Nantais & Kuczewksi, 2004). Involving the patient in the decision means that the patient can analyze his or her quality of life, based on the goals the patient had hoped to achieve before the illness.

This highlights the concept that in the United States, medical treatment is based on informed consent. Basically, informed consent means that an individual has the right to refuse medical treatment that he or she does not believe will contribute to his or her well-being. My diabetic patient is a prime example of informed consent. However, if a patient can't make that decision because of unsoundness of mind, others might be asked. These "others" are those closest to a patient, like a spouse, sibling, or parent. Many times, these health care "proxies" are asked to make medical treatment decisions when the patient can't. The assumpion here is that after the patient, the proxy has the best understanding of what's in the patient's best interests.

While studies show that third parties might rate the patient's QOL lower than the patient, this is different when it comes to end-of-life scenarios. In these situations, proxies do a reasonable job of guessing the patient's wishes.

So how did Michael Schiavo fail so miserably as Terri's proxy? No, she didn't leave any kind of advanced directive, but as her spouse, Michael should have known his wife's wishes. He even said, at one point, that Terri indicated she didn't want to survive as a vegetable. He had the right to remove his wife's feeding tube. After all, it isn't as though he suggested it be removed at once. The decision was made only after years of various standard and experimental therapies that proved to be ineffective.

The challenge was that Terri's parents never accepted the diagnosis of PVS and, as a result, resisted their son-in-law's decision to refuse life-sustaining measures on her behalf. How could she be a vegetable? Didn't she react to Mary Schindler's voice? Didn't she laugh, cry, and moan? Did her eyes follow a red balloon around the room? Didn't all that show that she was aware?

From a medical standpoint, the answer is no. But from the standpoint of the parents, Terri was still in there, somewhere. Sadly, the ongoing court battle and the battle in the court of public opinion only served to muddy the waters.

Quality of Life Versus Health

When people lose money or material goods, they might shrug and say "at least I have my health." But does health necessarily mean happiness?

Health can be considered a physical and psychological ability to fulfill basic needs when it comes to functioning in basic social roles (Musschenga, 1997). However, health, in and of itself, doesn't necessarily always lead to happiness (Musschenga, 1997).

Going further, quality of life and happiness can be linked, but QOL differs from individual to individual. For instance, a soccer star who loses his leg in an accident will never be able to play soccer on the same level (Musschenga, 1997). This could be devastasting to the player; to him, soccer is life. This player might want to die, because without his ability to play soccer, life has no meaning.

However, a professor who loses a leg in a similar accident might have another outlook. Certainly, living his life will require an adjustment with a prosthesis or wheelchair, but it won't stop him when it comes to doing what he likes, which is teaching and research. He can continue to build a good quality of life, doing what he loves to do.

The takeaway from all of this is there is no such thing

as a single viewpoint when it comes to quality of life. While medicine still has its focus on Cartesian dualism, there is some evidence that the important thing here isn't that all life is sacred, no matter the quality.

In many cases, medicine is doing its best to help those with chronic conditions live as comfortably as possible. Treatment decisions tend to be based on a level of human functionality. Will the patient be able to function independently? What are the life goals of the patient and how might medical treatment impact those goals?

Above all, doctors are starting to listen to patients and those who know them best when dealing with quality of life issues. In some cases, like the situation with my diabetic patint, they aren't forcing the issue when the patient decides that the time for treatment ends, and it's time to go.

Additionally, while the Terri Schiavo case generated heartbreak and sensationalism, it also increased awarenes of issues like written advanced directives and do-not-rescuitate orders. All of this provides individuals with more power over their quality of life—and when treatments should no longer be necessary.

PART 3
WHERE WE NEED TO BE

❋ Getting Philosophy Back into Medicine

Let's review.

PHILOSOPHY CONCERNS THE STUDY OF CERtain questions, generally about existence and the reason for life. Medicine focuses on procedures and practices used to treat or prevent diseases. Though they appear to be separate, these two concepts went hand-in-hand, at least, until the Age of Reason, when advances in science and dualism came into play.

Yet philosophical existentialism and concepts of mind/body/soul can work quite well with medicine. In fact, within today's medical practices, philosophy is an important concept. Before determining how these two fit together, let's get back to ancient Greece, Aristotle, and his virtue ethics.

Defining Virtue—and Ethics

From Aristotle's point of view, virtue ethics supported excellence in both reason and character in humankind. In the practice of ancient medicine, as well as the practice of Western medicine today, virtue ethics means that a doctor or any other healthcare professional should exhibit compassion and honesty, along with morally correct actions in decision-making (Taylor, n.d.).

That's a large responsibility. It's also pretty vague. In Aristotle's time, healthcare decision-making was straightforward. If someone had an incurable disease, he or she died. Otherwise, medicine was in place to ensure that the patient could count on an ideal quality of life, or at least a relatively comfortable one until it came time to die.

The incurable diseases that plagued ancient Greeks (and pretty much everyone through the early part of the twentieth century) can be treated or prevented. Furthermore, people who would have died in BCE Greece can now be kept alive, whether their conscious mind is present or not. Doctors are morally correct in that they're not going to kill patients out of the blue, at least, assuming the doctor isn't an insane murderer. Even the "right-to-die" champion, Dr. Jack Kervorkian, though nicknamed "Dr. Death," didn't go around killing all terminal patients.

The question of "morality" becomes a little blurred when it comes to situations like end-of-life issues.

One doctor might be okay with disconnecting life support from a brain-dead patient. She might believe that this patient is, for all intents and purposes, dead (which technically is what brain death means). Keeping that patient alive on a ventilator would prolong the family's agony and use up healthcare and other resources that could benefit another patient. In fact, the majority of the medical profession supports disconnection of life support under these circumstances, understanding that no patient comes back from being brain dead. Comatose, yes. Brain dead? Absolutely not. Ultimately, the decision to end life support is up to the patient's proxy and family. Doctors can only go so far to encourage this kind of decision.

Yet there are a handful of doctors who actually view withholding of life support as a flagrant violation of a patient's right to live (Rajshekahr, et., al, 2017). They believe that it's also a violation of patient autonomy. These doctors might also subscribe to the belief that where there's life, there's hope. Again, that final decision isn't up to these doctors. Still, they can do their best to convince family members that there are reasons to continue treatment.

Terri Schiavo wasn't brain dead, yet many believed

that she wouldn't come out of her PVS. This meant a gray area concerning whether to keep the PEG tube in place or to remove it.

In the early days and years following Schiavo's collapse, her husband did everything he could to help her regain consciousness, including transporting her to California to have experimental electrodes placed into her brain (Wolfson, 2006). This followed years of physical and occupational therapy in attempts to rehabilitate her. Michael Schiavo finally understood that nothing more could be done, and that his wife would simply not recover. She was brain damaged. Michael Schiavo believed that Terri would not have wanted to survive in a minimal vegetative state.

Yet her parents never accepted the PVS diagnosis. They believed that Terri would come out of it and get back to normal. They pointed to her "responsiveness." They kept hope going (not to mention the courts) until the feeding tube was finally removed and Terri died. Through the lens of virtue ethics, both sides were technically right. No one wanted to cause Terri pain. Both sides believed that their views and actions could help Terri live her best life.

In cases that are less extreme than Schiavo's, what does virtue ethics mean? The concept of morally correct decision-making is pretty broad for the doctor. What might be the right treatment path for one patient might not necessarily be effective for another. In all cases, it's in the doctor's best interest to provide the best options for patients. Again, the power should be in the patient's hands to determine the best path forward.

Utilitarianism and Deontology—Society Versus Person

Unlike the relative vagueness of virtue ethics, utilitarianism is pretty clear-cut in its aims. Specifically, utilitarianism believes that decisions should be made to benefit the most people. A utilitarian viewpoint of the Schiavo case would have been clear-cut: Schiavo, with her damaged brain, was taking up medical resources that could benefit other patients who might have more positive outcomes.

I mentioned earlier in this paper that the practice of medicine today doesn't necessarily mesh with philosophy. If there is any philosophical belief that matches the medical practice of today, it's utilitarianism.

Medical resources are scarce. They also are costly. Under utilitarian philosophy, doctors and other health-care professionals (as well as insurance companies) make treatment decisions based on what is likely to provide the best benefit to the most people.

Evidence-based medicine could also fit under the utilitarian philosophy. It supports the idea that treatments benefitting populations should be used with various patients because they were proven to work. There doesn't need to be costly or time-consuming experimentation with other types of treatment.

Incidentally, utilitarianism could be why the pharmaceutical industry researches and develops drugs to benefit vast swaths of the population suffering from mainly chronic illnesses. There's the profit motiviation, of course. But there's also the idea that many people can benefit from a particular drug or group of drugs.

Unfortunately, this means that individuals with rare diseases lose out. Let's put it this way. You can find a lot of drugs out there to treat cholesterol and hypertension. (You can also learn about these drugs through the incessant advertising created by Big Pharma.) When it comes to the more rare disease of glioblastoma multiforme (GBM), a type of brain tumor, the options are more limited.

This is because around 12,000 cases of GBM are diagnosed in the United States in a given year. Compare this to the ninety-four million adults who experience high cholesterol annually. Even though Senators John McCain and Edward Kennedy both were diagnosed and died from GBM, this disease doesn't impact as many people as the scourge of high cholesterol. From Big Pharma's point of view, there's more money to be earned from ninety-four million adults versus 12,000 people. In addition to profit motives, this viewpoint is utilitarianism at its best.

On the opposite side of utilitarianism is deontology. Introduced by Immauel Kant, deontology is focused more on specific obligations or principles. From a healthcare perspective, deontological thinkers view the practice of medicine as a long-term relationship rather than the one-and-done that can be the typical stance of many doctors. In fact, deontological doctors fuly believe that the patient-physician relationship is just as important, if not more so, than physical treatment when it comes to dealing with disease and quality of life.

For instance, it's true that there aren't many treatment options for GBM. The disease is invariably fatal, with death occurring (in most cases) anywhere between twelve and eighteen months after diagnosis. However, there are many ongoing clinical trials involved with extending the life of those with GBM. GBM patients can participate in these trials. During the process, the patient builds a close relationship with the doctor or doctors involved with the trial or trials. Over time, the GBM patient goes from being a number (or an object-body) to becoming a human being with hopes, dreams, pain, suffering, and concerns (live-body).

To sum all of this up from the perspective of medical treatment, utilitarianism is more concerned with which outcomes generate the greatest benefit for the most number of people. Deontology, on the other hand, offers more of a patient-centered viewpoint and approach.

Principalism—The Specific Philosophy of Medicine

Unlike deontology and utilitarianism, principalism is a philosophy specifically geared toward science and biomedical ethics (Beauchamp & Rauprich, 2016). The concept was introduced by Tom Beauchamp and James Childress, and relies on four basic ethical principles, some of which have already been mentioned (Beauchamp & Rauprich, 2016).

> *Respect for autonomy*: The physican must disclose medical and treatment options so the patient can determine the best path. This also supports informed consent, confidentiality, and honesty (or truth-telling). We're

no longer living in the days in which doctors kept bad news from patients. Under this ethical principle, the doctor assumes that the patient wants to know the news.

Nonmaleficence: This is the obligation not to inflect harm on others. You might remember this from the Hippocratic maxim *primum non nocrere*, or "first do no harm." "Harm" can consist of many issues, and not just physical ones. It means avoiding negligence in care. It also means that each medical action is weighed against the benefits, risks, and consequences. This isn't too far off from the philosophy of consequentialism, which was discused above.

Beneficence: This is the physician's obligation to make decisions that benefit the patient. This also considers moral rules necessary to defend and protect the rights of others, remove conditions that could cause harm, and rescue those who might be in danger. It also encompasses the idea of acting in the best intersts of the patient.

Justice: All patients should qualify for equal treatment, in other words, a fair and equitable distribution of health resources. Racism or implicit biases, for example, have no place in healthcare delivery or treatment.

Principalism came about precisely to tackle moral situations in bioethics. The theory provides answers to situations in which there might be moral confusion about an issue. It also comes into play when two or more obligations are in place and only one can be met (Beauchamp & Rauprich, 2016). It provides a common language and response to ethical conflicts and issues that can arise in healthcare.

When used correctly, principalism can help guide highly difficult end-of-life decisions. It can also be useful in dealing with issues like dementia. It encompasses respect for autonomy, while also recognizing that care should be provided in conjunction with beneficence, justice, and nonmaleficence.

Principalism in the Real World

Let's examine a medical case study where principalism might be at work.

I've already indicated that the Jehovah's Witness faith

preaches against use of blood transfusions. Let's say that an unconscious twenty-five-year-old woman, a devout Jehovah's Witness, is admitted to a hospital after a car accident (Abimbola, 2013). She carries a card that confirms her objection to blood transfusions on religious grounds. Without that blood transfusion, though, the doctors can't perform surgery that would possibly save her life. The patient's mother, who is not of the Jehovah's Witness faith, insists on the blood transfusion.

From a utilitarian standpoint, the doctors would need to analyze the treatments necessary to maximize well-being in this situation. This might mean authorizing the transfusion because it would bring well-being to the mother. A virtue ethicist would focus on traits like generosity, trust, or ambivalence. Again, this might mean that the mother's wishes would be followed. The deontologist would make the decision by a moral rule, or the principal of autonomy. In this case, the doctors might honor the daughter's wishes, citing autonomy and decision-making.

Finally, if this young woman was admitted to a Western hospital adhering to the four principles of principalism, the focus would be on respect for autonomy (not to mention the need for fully informed consent). Nonmaleficence involves not inflicting harm on others. If the daughter had the transfusion and survived the surgery,

that could impact her negatively from a mental or emotional standpoint. Beneficence—acting in the best interest of the patient—means following the patient's wishes.
Finally, justice means getting rid of implicit bias. Even if
the doctors might want to authorize the blood transfusion
(and surgery), justice means that they will, once again,
follow the will of the patient.

Likely as not, this means the doctors wouldn't authorize the blood tranfusion, no matter the mother's
demands. Using this brand of philosophy, doctors go
beyond Cartesian dualism and simply treating illnesses.
Instead, they can provide options and treatments that
operate holistically, and that benefit not just a patient's
physical being, but the patient's well-being, too.

Culture and Healthcare

While all ethical points of principalism are important, one that tends to have the greatest focus is justice,
or equitable distribution of healthcare. This can involve
culture; when it comes to certain cultures and ethnicities,
the equitable distribution of healthcare can be a large
question mark.

But what is culture? Culture is defined as learned
behavior, both among members of a group and between

generations in a particular group (Berlinger & Berlinger, 2017). Culture can also be a distress code in conjunction with medical treatment and healthcare. We can see this, especially when religion enters into the situation. Jehovah's Witnesses regularly refuse blood products. Christian Scientists also forgo most medical treatments, belieiving that their own faith is sufficient to prevent illness and cure disease.

It could be said that culture was at work even with the fight over removing Terri Schiavo's feeding tube. The nationwide battle (and even the political battle) encompassed two camps: right to life and death with dignity. Those supporting Terri's right to live supported that right on religious grounds: the idea that all life is sacred, no matter the quality.

Out of the media limelight, culture, religion, and race tend to be set aside in certain healthcare situations. We saw this during the COVID-19 pandemic. The virus had a disproportionate impact on racial and ethnic groups, including African Americans, Native Americans and Hispanic/LatinX communities (Tai, Shah, Doubeni, Sia, & Wieland, 2021).

There were several reasons for this. Minority groups, overall, tend to have less access to healthcare, which might have led to worse COVID symptoms (and death).

Members of minority communities were also more likely to work in jobs that led to a higher risk of exposure. There is also the overall distrust of the healthcare profession, created by decades of bias and prejudice.

Because of this, minority groups were less likely to receive COVID vaccines than their white counterparts. There tended to be less access to the vaccines. Furthermore, there was a vast amount of institutional distrust, not to mention a lot of misinformation floating around.

Some of that institutional distrust isn't misplaced. Doctors can issue confusing treatment orders; even patients who are well-read and who have a relative understanding of disease and treatment can be baffled by such pronouncements. Additionally, doctors also tend to make decisions based on implicit bias, assumptions, and even stereotypes when it comes to treating patients.

Here's an example. A couple of ways to treat blood pressure are with dietary and lifestyle changes and medication. This is the treatment plan issued to people of all cultures and ethnicities. However, let's say that a doctor suggests this treatment plan to an African American woman, only to find that the patient hasn't been taking her pills, increasing her physical activity, or losing weight. The doctor (assuming he is a white male) might assume that the patient is just being stubborn.

This could be. Maybe the patient likes her weight just fine and doesn't want to deal with pills. It might not have anything to do with stubborness at all.

Maybe in the patient's cultural background, food is highly important. It's an important part of socialization and community. In fact, in this particular culture, failure to eat could be a sign of something wrong, leading to all kinds of unwelcome questions from friends and family.

Maybe the patient isn't being difficult when it comes to improving her activity. This lack could be a result of her environment. If she lives in a lower-income area, it might not be safe to walk, due to traffic or other concerns. She also doesn't have the disposable income to take part in other types of exercise, like joining a fitness center.

What about failure to take medicine? This could result from a couple of factors. First is not understanding why the pills are necessary in the first place. Second could be finances. That patient might not have the funds to buy the prescrption drugs, and pride might stop her from saying anything to her doctor.

Instead of understanding cultural nuances, however, a doctor might be more likely to lecture this "noncompliant" patient in hopes that a good talking to will result in some action. Rather than moving this patient toward better compliance, that lecture will result in shame and anger. This could mean a higher level of noncompliance. If the patient is noncompliant for a long enough period, her high cholesterol could lead to a heart attack or stroke. This means hospitalization, and more strain on already scarce healthcare resources.

Rather than yelling at someone for not taking the blood pressure medicine on a regular basis, it's better if the doctor can understand and anticipate the cultural, ethnic, and sociological drivers that underlie that decision. There could be a genuine antipathy toward pills of any kind. Maybe language barriers are preventing a true understanding of how and why taking the pills is important.

❈ The Philosophy of Medicine: Its Very Own Field

The common theme of this paper is that for a good part of the twentieth century, the pratice of medicine involved a focus on body-as-object. The mind and emotions were considered separate and apart, while the patient rarely, if ever, had a say in his or her care or diagnosis. In many cases, this is the situation today.

However, things are changing. Actually, that change began in the late 1990s, possibly as one of the managed-care backlashes. Alternative medicine moved from the "woo and wacky" margins to hesitantly merge with mainstream medicine. Acupuncture is sometimes suggested for pain, and many hospitals are incorporating trained aromatherpists to aid with patient relaxation.

Additionally, proponents of medical education are stressing the need to do more than teach anatomy and physiiology. They regularly make the case for holistic medical care and education (Mantri, 2008). This isn't totally eliminating Cartesian dualism, however. We're still dealing with a healthcare system that focuses on costs and standardized diagnoses. There has, however, been a subtle shift from the mind/body/soul separation (Arnaudo, 2017). This is how things should be. Medicine should go beyond just a body focus and "parts" specialization, and focus on treating—and healing—the entire individual.

Here's another interesting trend. Philosophy of medicine is becoming a field of its own. In my discussion concerning the history of medicine, I stated that the *Hippocratic Corpus*, among other sources, entwined philosophy and medicine/science. These days, the specific philosophy of medicine field offers a lot of information, including dedicated journals, professional organizations, and a growing base of scholarly literature (Reiss, 2016).

Here's the downside. Just like defining medicine and philosophy (separately), the philosophy of medicine is a hugely broad field. Reiss defines this concept as an exploration of the basic and fundamental issues in theory, practice, and research within the health sciences.This, in turn, encompasses not just physiology and treatment, but non-physical issues, like metaphysics and epistemology.

Meanwhile, Tosam (2014) suggests that the philsophy of medicine represents a philosopical analysis of medical issues, disease, health, and care. As such, the aspects of medicine and healthcare delivery go beyond the physical nature of disease or illness.

Then there is the idea that the philosophy of medicine means that philosophical approaches become instruments and methods to help generate knowledge about medicine. This is opposed to using medicine as a jumping-off point to gain knowledge about philosophical methods and approaches (Schramme, 2015). In other words, it is the difference between using medical examples to philisoph-ically discuss or analyze pain versus analyzing suffering relative to the goals of medicine.

Confused yet? Keep reading.

In referencing Henrick Wulff (1992), William Stempsey (2008) points out that practitioners in this field include:

- Professional philosophers who are interested in medical matters;
- Physicians who have a deep interest in philosophy;
- Professional philosophers who are well-versed in medicine;
- Medical professionals who are trained in philosophy; and
- Medical professionals who devote themselves to medical pratice.

In some ways, all of the practitioners listed above formulate problems within, and contribute to, the philosophy of medicine (Stempsey, 2008; Wulff, 1992).

To make the situation a little more clear, let's try to narrow down the definition. The philosophy of medicine goes beyond the physical "medical" treatment to determine other areas important to identifying and maintaining the health and well-being of patients. It covers issues like causation of an illness or disease, the patient-physical relationship, and the mind-body interaction that supports treatment. As such, philosophy of medicine goes beyond just curing disease or illnesses. The goals of this concept are to

1. Make the patient an active partner in his or her healthcare and medical treatment; and

2. Do what's needed to help that patient reach his or her own path to health and quality of life.

The main point of this definition is that it's individualistic. It doesn't tell us what quality of life should be. Rather, it makes the patient a participant in developing the right QOL to suit that particular patient. Rather than putting the doctor at the center of treatment, it allows the patient in as a partner.

This concept also supports the basis of self-healing, an essential situation for any human being. Understanding the philosophy of medicine also means being familiar with, and understanding, the terminology involved with it. Here are some modes of philosophical thought that are part and parcel of this field.

Reductionism: Divide, Divide, and Conquer

Reductionism isn't too different from the Cartesian dualism that's part of Western medical practice. Both reductionism and dualism divide complex objects into their smallest parts. Yes, those "complex objects" mean human beings. Going another step further, metaphysical reductionism, also known as ontological reductionism, separates those parts, creating even smaller parts (Marcum, n.d.).

Here's a familiar refrain: Reductionists believe that bodies are machines, with disease the result of a mechanical dysfunction at the genetic and even molecular level (Tosam, 2014). Here's something else that's also familiar: Reductionism tends to support medical specialization.

In today's practice of medicine, reductionism indicates how a biomedical scientist might investigate and explain a disease, as well as how a clinician might diagnose and treat it (Marcum, n.d.).

Reductionism asks a single question when it comes to treatments and medical care: "Can a disease be sufficiently reduced to its elemental components?" For example, if a biomedical researcher believes that brain process dysfunction is the cause of mental or emotional illness, that reseacher will look at it from a molecular level. From there, the researcher might find a lack of serotonin, a neurotransmitter, is the cause for mental and emotional issues. The researcher then might come up with a chemical compound to improve serotonin levels. This moves on to the clinician, who diagnoses a patient's depression in terms of a seratonin lack, and then prescribes the appropriate antidepressant to deal with the issue (Marcum, n.d.).

I've already discussed at length the problems and challenges with Cartesian dualism. Because reductionism is similar, the same challenges exist. Reductionism—well, it reduces. It forgets that the human body is a complex, interconnected system rather than the sum of its parts. By complex system, I mean the physical aspects that keep it running. I also mean the non-physical parts, including life experiences, environment, beliefs, spirituality, and so on.

Holism: The Entire Enchilada

Holism is the exact opposite of reductionism. Rather than dividing into parts, and then dividing those parts into even more parts, holism likes to look at the forest rather than the trees (to coin an infamous old adage). When it comes to treating disease and illness, a holistic practioner will look at the physical issues as well as other issues. Holism is the view that parts of the whole are connected and related to one another (Tosam, 2014). Holists regard the patient as an entire being, rather than a combination of parts that can be measured or calculated.

With the above example concerning the patient who suffers from a brain process dysfunction, a holist won't deny that a lack of serotonin might be one of the causes. The clinician working with that patient might also examine other factors. She might consider the patient's living situation, environment, diet, and other issues. She might take a look at the patient's overall family dynamics and even ask about the culture. The resulting treatment plan might include an antidepressant prescription. The clinician might also suggest that the patient stay away from refined sugar, schedule a daily walk in her schedule, and even practice some mindfulness meditation.

Here's another example, one dealing with a physical issue. Let's say a patient ends up with a diagnosis of leukemia. The reductionist doctor will measure white blood cells and red blood cells in connection with regular chemotherapy. When the white blood cell and red blood cell counts are within range, the reductionist doctor and the patient go their separate ways.

The holistic doctor also considers the blood cell counts and prescribes chemotherapy. The holistic doctor might also examine the patient's family history to determine if there's a genetic predisposition. The doctor will also monitor the patient's emotional health (cancer can be a shock to the emotional and mental system). The doctor might also keep an eye on any side effects the chemo generates, and determine solutions to reduce some of the worst ones. Once the cancer is in remission, the holistic doctor will suggest that the patient continue to follow up.

To summarize, the reductionist's goal is to pinpoint

the disease, treat it, and send the patient home. However, the holistic doctor will go beyond just looking at the disease. Rather than eradication as the goal, this doctor will determine both the disease and what it might mean to a patient's overall life and well-being.

Realism Versus Anti-Realism

Reductionism and holism are straightforward philosophy of medicine topics. However, realism and anti-realism can muddy the philosophic waters.

Realism (in terms of philosophy of medicine) means that objects and events are independent of the person observing them (Marcum, n.d.). In other words, things will go on being—well, things, whether or not we are actively observing them.

Let's step outside the medical field for a moment to analyze another adage, the one about the tree falling in the woods. The specific question is, if no one is around, will that falling tree make a sound? To the realist, the answer is yes. That tree will make a sound when it falls, whether or not anyone is around. This is because it's assumed that falling trees are noisy, whether people are in earshot or not.

On a scientific level, we know that bacteria and cells

exist in the natural world, but they don't require human minds to prove they exist. We just know they're there.

Let's get back to our patient with the brain processing dysfunction/depression. If a doctor steeped in realism is treating this individual, he understands that seratonin already exists in the brain, even if it can't be seen by the naked eye (nor is it under observation 24/7). Because he knows that a lack of the neurotransmitter might be causing a problem (even if he can't see it), the doctor's move might be to treat the patient using anti-depressant or other medications. The outcome that the realist doctor wants to achieve is eradication, or absence, of the depression.

Anti-realism takes another tack. Instead of assuming that things exist (even if we can't always see or observe them), the philosophical belief of the anti-realist is that observable objects and events are highly dependent on the person observing them. Getting back to the question of our falling tree, the anti-realist's immediate response isn't "of course it makes a noise, all the time." Instead, the anti-realist would say that it depends. If someone is in the woods while the tree is falling, then yes, it makes a sound. If no one is around, however, there is no noise. This is because no one is around to observe the action.

To apply this to the medical field, not all bacteria or cells are real, but rather, are specific constructs. If we're talking about the patient with depression, the above-mentioned serotonin isn't real at all to an anti-realism physician, but rather, it is "a laboratory or clinical construct based on experimental or clincial conditionsly balancing serotonin levels, especialy as the neurtransmitter is more of a construct" (Tosam, 2014). The treatment might involve other tools to help the patient feel better.

Metaphysics and Epistemology: Being or Knowing?

Mention the term *metaphysics* and the first things that might come to mind are the supernatural and the occult. In the area of philosophy, however, metaphysics focuses on non-visible and non-measurable factors, with a focus on the nature of an object's existence and potential connected forces.

More to the point, metaphysics is a branch of philosophy concering itself with the nature of reality. It can also mean "beyond" nature, involving things that might not be immediately visible or even measurable. Metaphysics, above all, is a cause-and-effect phliosophy, concerning itself with the causes of both health and disease and, as the basis of this involves matter, consciousness and even spirit.

Meanwhile, there's ontology, which is a branch of

metaphysics. Ontology delves further into the meaning of existence (or rather, what does or doesn't exist). Ontology is sometimes considered the "science of being" in that its focus is on both the nature of objects and how their forces connect. It shouldn't come as much of a surprise that metaphysics and ontology tend to be important when it comes to understanding both disease and health.

While ontology can be considered the doctrine of being, epistemology is more along the lines of the doctrine of knowing or theory. Basically, epistemology concerns itself specifically with human knowledge, its nature, origin, and scope, and the reliability of claims to knowledge. Rather than strict cause-and-effect, as with both metaphysics and ontology, epistemology attempts to answer questions like "What is the source of our knowledge?" or "What is its structure and what are its limits?" Other important questions include "How do we know that we know?" and "What are the necessary and sufficient conditions for knowledge?"

One epistemological problem is medical uncertainty. Though many Western doctors might disagree, medical knowledge is highly uncertain. It's also imperfect and incomplete. This is obvious with even just a casual glance at the history of medicine and healthcare. Under epistemology, this uncertainty can be mitigated in a few ways, one of which is sharing the decision-making responsibility with a patient or even consulting with other clinicians to obtain their viewpoints on a particular disease or treatment.

Causality—and Outcomes

Dualism and reductionism tend to reduce the human body, and disease, to its various parts. Causality introduces a different wrinkle into the situation. The most common causality can be summed up as "if A happens, then B will occur." This isn't all that different from the above-mentioned consequentialism, in which certain actions will result in specific outcomes. Causality is also an important concept when it comes to philosophy of medicine.

We can trace causality all the way back to Aristotle, who indicated four causal categories. They are

- Material, or what something is made of, or from;
- Formal, or how something is made;
- Efficiency, or what forces are responsible for making something; and
- Final cause, the reason, or end purpose why something is made. (Tosam 2014, page number)

During the seventeenth century, Frances Bacon reduced the four to two: material and efficiency. Meanwhile, David Hume eschewed the idea of causality. In the world of dualism medicine, causality exerts its influence—a disease might occur because of a specific physical or chemical reason.

Here's a common causal statement: Cigarettes cause lung cancer. There's the cause (cigarettes) and the effect (lung cancer). But this tie-in isn't so much cause and effect as it is epidemological evidence. Certainly, a high percentage of lung cancers can be attributed to smoking, but non-smokers can also develop lung cancer. Furthermore, many cigarette smokers go through life without getting this horrific disease.

Most times, causality is less "philosophical" and more "scientific." This is because the physical-disease causality is mainly a biological issue. This is all well and good, but it also ignores the fact that someone can be ill or in pain without actually suffering from tissue damage or a disease.

The advent of philosophy of medicine represents a positive step forward for healthcare. Though all of the philosophical principles aren't perfect, the field is opening the discussion beyond just science, physiology, and anatomy. Philosophy of medicine is starting to provoke the questions concerning not just disease treatment but overall healing as well.

⚜ Mind-Body for Healing

EBM versus PCM

Before moving forward, let's get back to the idea of Evidence-Based Medicine. To reiterate, EBM allows doctors and clinicians to base their medical decisions and practices on the best available scientific and clinical evidence. EBM makes sense, to a point. When it comes to certain patients and disease, using already proven clinical evidence can help take the guesswork out of diagnosis and treatment.

However, EBM eschews pathphysiology, with its focus on how body function changes due to the disease process. It also tends to ingore the doctor's personal experience, or "gut" feeling. Another concept mentioned in this paper is that the practice of medicine is actually an art. EBM also doesn't agree with this. It should comes as no surprise that EBM slots nicely into the Cartesian dualism practice of today's Western medicine.

Then there is patient-centered medicine. This is sometimes known as person-centered medicine or PCM. While

EBM provides a vast pool of data from which a doctor or clinician can choose for help with diagnosis and treatment, PCM is more focused on the patient and the patient's personal information. Once that information is collected and analyzed (with the patient as a willing participant), the doctor is able to determine the best and most effective treatment for that particular patient (Marcum, n.d.).

Basically, PCM suggests that medicine should reintroduce what the discipline forgot during its focus on empricism: that the patient is a situated, social, and relational human being (Kirkengen, et al., 2016). This also involves a mind-body connection when it comes to medical treatment. PCM focuses instead on the patient's experience with the disease, and seeks methods to mitigate pain or discomfort.

In a previous chapter, I introduced the story of an African American female who was diagnosed with high cholesterol. We pointed out that EBM might suggest that certain statins can help in lowering the "bad" numbers. In this particular situation, the woman didn't take her pills or participate in any of the lifestyle changes suggested by the doctor.

If that doctor had practiced PCM, he would have actively discussed what the patient might be able to do. If walking was out of the question (due to being in a neighborhood that might not allow that exercise), the doctor could have discussed at-home or at-work exercises for her. Diet change might also have been an issue. From a PCM standpoint, the doctor could have made suggestions as to how she could still partake of food and socialization while looking after her health. It's possible that if this woman felt like the doctor was on her side instead of lecturing her about taking pills, she might have been less stressed and more compliant when it came to taking charge of her own treatment. She might have suffered from less stress in the process of pulling herself to better health.

The Brain, Stress, and Total Healing

Talk of stress brings us to talk about the brain. While the brain is one of the most active organs of the human body, we unfortunately don't know a whole lot about it. We do understand that this organ is responsible for human maintenance (Bhat, Parr, Ramstead, & Friston, 2021). When the brain dies, so does the body.

We also know that the brain is in contact with the immune system, 24/7, 365 days a year This communication ensures that brain and immune system share the same goal, which is to protect the body from harm by distinguishing "threats" and "non-threats." Furthermore, the brain and body are in constant communication, authorizing an ongoing, multidirectional flow of information consisting of hormones, neurotransmitters, and cytokines (Vitetta, Anton, Cortizo, & Sali, 2005).

Going one step further, there has been plenty of research explaining that stress can have a definite impact on physical functioning and brain functioning. Stress can lead to problems with neural circuitry, resulting in mood changes and increases in anxiety. This, in turn, can actively impact an individual's behavior.

Because of the brain's connection with the body, it's important to understand the role of stress in all types of functioning. A 1980s study among women with breast cancer noted that stress reduction and social support as a therapeutic intervention to illness could help alleviate physical issues (Brower, 2006). In recent years, other studies among workers in low-level jobs that generated high stress showed that this stress led to physical issues like metabolic syndrome. This, in turn, can be a a precursor of heart disease and diabetes.

Thanks to this and other research, the medical profession has been more open to the idea that negative life stressors and unhappy emotional states can have an impact on bodily functions (Vitetta, Anton, Cortizo, & Sali, 2005). But this wasn't always the situation.

Dean Ornish, clinical professor at the University of California-San Francisco and founder, president, and director of the Preventative Medicine Research Institute, introduced the holistic viewpoint. He connected the idea that helping to eliminate stress and improve lifestyle could lead to positive results among those who had, or were at risk of, heart disease (Brower, 2006). As far back as the 1980s, he postulated that heart disease could be managed and reversed with simple lifestyle changes including exercise and weight loss. He also noted that "non-medical" tools, like meditation or yoga, stress management, and social support could also be helpful in reducing stress and putting the patient into a more positive frame of mind.

But Ornish was laughed at. Why? Because this was a period of time during which heart disease was treated the old-fashioned way: through pills and surgical procedures like bypass and angioplasty. Heart transplants for truly non-working hearts were also in play. Ornish had the last laugh. During the past several decades, scientific research and numerous studies have been done on lifestyle change and their impact on heart disease. You probably know what's coming next. Ornish's methods were proven viable in treating heart disease. In fact, Ornish's program has been adopted by many cardiologists and cardiovascular clinics to great success.

This is one example about what Western medicine needs to do to help a patient truly heal from whatever ails. The common theme here is that, to help a patient heal, the doctor needs to address more than physiology and anatomy. She also needs to regard the patient under the lived-body lens. This involves the following.

1. Understanding the physical disease, illness or condition that brought the patient to the doctor in the first place; and
2. How this disease, illness or condition is impacting the patient's mind, body, emotions and spirit. (Karff, 2009).

Remember the earlier example where you went to the doctor because of a stomach ache, and the doctor's response was to hand you a bottle of pills and refer you to a specialist? Here's a potential change. Instead of the pills and the referral, the doctor sat down with you and asked you specifically when the pain started, what was going on in your life before hand, and if there just might be a connection. It's possible that you might still get the prescription and might have to pay a visit to a gastro-enterologist. It could also be that the doctor might give you anti-anxiety medication and suggest that you take up yoga or meditation (assuming, of course, that there's no evidence of a specific issue, like a burst appendix or ulcer).

So what seems to be driving the mellowing of Western medicine? Some of it has to do with greater demand on the part of patients for a higher degree of autonomy and decision-making when it comes to their care (Brower, 2006). Furthermore, today's patients are better-educated, thanks to the internet. Rather than asking a doctor what ails, they might actually introduce their own opinions.

As an aside, some doctors don't like this, partly because it puts their own expertise into question, and partly because there is a huge chance of misdiagnosis. The point here is that patients are working hard to take charge of their own health.

There is also a growing dissatisfaction with allopathic medicine when treating and preventing chronic illnesses (Brower, 2006). Some people simply don't want to swallow pills to control cholesterol or blood pressure. They're afraid of the side effects. They don't want more chemicals in their body than what the environment is already providing. Furthermore, given the ridiculous costs of drugs, some patients might view traditional medicines as too expensive.

These patients might think there's a more natural way to reduce blood pressure and cholesterol, and are going the alternative medicine route. In the early 1990s, when the National Institutes of Health opened its Office of Alternative Medicine, more than one-third of Americans said they used relaxation techniques and imagery, biofeedback, and hypnosis to help achieve healing and health. Additionally, more than 50 percent of them indicated they use prayer as a complementary or alternative therapy.

While the internet can be responsible for a lot of misinformation, it also helps patients gain the right kind of knowledge, knowledge which was once the sole province of the medical "gatekeepers." When patients can speak to doctors in this language and properly delineate their symptoms, this increases their cultural health capital. They aren't quite so willing to accede meekly to a specialist referral or prescription. Rather, they'll ask questions and want outcomes.

This is a postive move forward in Western medicine. Even though Western medicine retains much of its "body-object" concept, patients aren't as willing to accept this. On the other side of the treatment barrier, doctors, too, are starting to understand that body and mind are interlinked, and need to be treated as a single unit rather than being separated. It is like that song about love and marriage: you can't have one without the other.

The Physician-Patient Relationship

Speaking of relationships, another important one is what's known as the "doctor-patient therapeutic alliance." Earlier in this paper, I listed many of the downsides of medicine without philosophical existentialism or thinking. To repeat, this type of medical practice can lead to more mistakes and a "disconnect" on the doctor's side. It can also lead to distrust, anxiety, and unhappiness from the patient's point of view.

As such, a positive doctor-patient relationship becomes supremely important in healthcare outcomes. This partnership was once taken for granted; for centuries, conventional wisdom was that there was healing power in a positive doctor-patient relationship (Karff, 2009). But by the middle of the twentieth century (thanks to medical technology and the cures of multiple diseases), healing depended only on the quality of the physician, the physician's education, and his or her knowledge. Furthermore, it didn't matter if a medical specialist had a good bedside manner. That specialist's job was simply to "cure" a patient. There was no need to become best friends with that individual.

These days, we're seeing research and articles that extol the virtues of a positive doctor-patient relationship.

The main reason is practical. Dislike of a doctor can directly impact a patient's ability to heal, for the following reasons (Selig, 2021).

- A patient is less likely to reveal symptoms and other important health issues to unsympathetic doctors;
- Doctors who operate on a less impersonal level are more prone to misdiagnoses;
- Doctors who come across as dismissive or uncaring could cause patients to neglect their own health;
- Patients who dislike their doctors are under stress, which can interfere with understanding medical information that is presented; and
- Patients are less likely to follow doctor recommendations if they're not able to ask follow-up questions about issues including side effects or outcomes.

The basic takeaway here is that both doctors and patients should move in the direction of having a positive relationship. I've already indicated a problem with this. In today's segmented healthcare delivery system, doctors might not have the time to build these positive relationships with their patients. I noted that the deadline orientation of healthcare delivery tends to reduce interactions between doctors and patients. This is a problem, as the therapeutic value of a commited doctor-patient relationship can lead to better outcomes.

One way in which this can be mitigated is through the use of technology. Thanks to various online platforms and an increase in telehealth, patients can ask questions of their doctors between visits and receive somewhat rapid responses. While this might not be an optimal form of relationship-building, it allows for back-and-forth communication if the patient has concerns.

Martin Heidegger—Medicine, Mind, and Body

Much of the above fits into the theories of another philosopher. Martin Heidegger was a twentieth-century German philosopher who was known for tying mind, body, and health together through his writings.

Before continuing, we need to point out that Heidegger was a controversial philosopher because of his ties to the Nazi Party (Wheeler, 2011). In this role, he helped implement Nazi educational and cultural programs in his native Freiburg. Whatever his politics, Heidegger did understand the importance of the mind-body connection in the pursuit of health (Boudreau, 2018).

In his writings (one of which was entitled *Being and Time*), Heidegger focused on the idea that a person in balance is "being-in-the-world." Doctors can support that balance through their skills and techne. But he also emphatically pointed out that medical skills should be in play to reveal truth.

However, he's best-known for discussing the lived experience of disease. Heidegger indicated that a patient with good health could be described as "homelikeness" and one in ill health as "unhomelikeness." A patient who is ill (unhomelikeness) views the world differently. The patient is disoriented; it takes effort to get things done. As such, Heidegger indicated that any medical care should consider how the patient views the world while he or she is ill.

Additionally, he stated that any medical skills used to support a patient's change required the doctor to understand the limitations of human condition. As such, health and well-being are not just the product of medical technology, but are also due to individual perception. Heidegger also supported the doctor-patient relationship, noting that the practice of healing is based on that particular partnership.

The Patient is (Rarely) Crazy

Heidegger's differences between "homelikeness" and "unhomelikeness" bring up another facet of a mind-body connection (and by extention, philosophy). As I've noted, during much of the nineteenth and twentieth centuries, if a person was ailing and a direct cause could be found, that cause was isolated and treated. Conversely, if a person was ill without a direct cause, that problem was considered to be in the person's head. What followed was a visit, or several visits, to a mental health professional, and an unfortunate stigma on that person's life. This became more of a stressful issue for the person when those visits didn't "cure" what ailed.

In his theories of "homelikeness" and "unhomelikeness," Heidegger explained that it isn't just a mental issue if someone is ill. If someone is genuinely not feeling well, whether there's a specific physical cause or not, this is aproblem, and it's up to the doctor to realize this. As I continually say in this paper, it's not just the disease or illness that's important; it's also how the patient reacts in the throes of not feeling well. Treatments must examine that as well.

Fortunately, there's a growing appreciation for mental, emotional, and lifestyle influences on physical well-being. In many cases, if a patient comes in with a complaint, and there's no evidence of illness or disease, a doctor might ask what's going on in this patient's life. Not all doctors do this, and we're nowhere near where we need to be when it comes to the holistic mind-body concept. But it's a start.

Interestingly enough, this is how medicine used to be practiced. Doctors working with patients before the age of Cartesian dualism strove to achieve a "homelikeness" when it came to health. That included anything and everything that might pertain to why a patient might ail. This is not to romanticize the medical past—there was plenty wrong with it. However, the key to a patient's health should be to combine yesteryear's doctor-patient relationship with today's medical technology and tools.

❋ Getting Back to "Start" Again

"The physician should not be afraid to engage in philosophical studies," said medical historian Henry E. Sigerist. "If he wants to be more than a narrow specialist, he must look at medicine from a wide perspective and must be aware of the place that medicine takes in our body of knowledge" (p. 162).

Sigerist isn't wrong. The question is whether this is happening. My assertion is that it's happening—slowly. Unfortunately, things keep occurring to put us back into the whole Cartesian dualism, object-body medical format.

Let's examine the recent COVID-19 pandemic and how that played out. At first, the doctors and other scientists couldn't figure out how the disease was transmitted.

In a world-wide effort, researchers banded together to determine the cells that generated the disease and how it was transmitted. This, in turn, led to requests for social distancing, mask-wearing, and not one but three types of vaccines that could at least arm the body against possible incursion of the virus. This was the science side of the situation.

In the end, COVID-19 killed more than one million people. We're still not out of the woods with it, as the disease is endemic. Continued research means more vaccines are being developed, enabling our bodies to better fight the virus. Thanks to this research, vaccines, and even medicines available for those who contract the disease, it's possible to survive it. We've come a long way from when COVID could be a death sentence.

Here's the next issue we're fighting: long COVID. Long COVID, sometimes referred to as "post-COVID conditions," describes the lingering symptoms of someone who was infected by the virus. Other names for Long COVID include long-haul COVD, post-acute COVID-19, long-term effects of COVID, or chronic COVID. Many of the symptoms include insomnia, smell and taste changes, shortness of breath, chest pain, palpitations, dizziness, depression, and anxiety (AMA, 2022). Sometimes, the symptoms are so debilitating, they interfere with a patient's quality of life. They aren't able to perform even normal daily activities.

Here's the problem. There isn't a specific cause related to Long COVID. There are some hypotheses—for example, it's possible that viral remnants in tissues is triggering inflammation, leading to problems. Another potential reason is autoimmunity from the disease. Even so, no one has really been able to put a finger on the cause.

Unfortunately, patients with Long COVID are experiencing the same disdain from the medical establishment as past patients did with disorders like chronic fatigue syndrome or fibromyalgia. Specifically, because there is no apparent reason for the multiple symptoms of Long COVID, doctors are ignoring it and turning their backs on it (Au, Capotescu, Eyal & Finestone, 2022). There are stories of patients who complain of symptoms being gaslit by the medical establishment. Rather than attempting to work with patients on what's wrong, these patients are dismissed.

Au, Capotescu, Eyal, and Finestone (2022) surmise that ontological politics is a main reason why Long COVID (and other non-causal disorders) tend to be dismissed rather than taken seriously. If there's no obvious cause, there's no specific relationship on which to hang a diagnosis. We get back to the idea that the patient has to prove his or her illness in order to gain access to any help from the medical community. In the finest example of medical gaslighting, these patients (especially woman and minorities) are not considered reliable reporters when it comes to their symptoms—or even their illnesses.

This can add stress to an already stressful situation. Let's put it this way: brain fog is no fun. It interferes with thinking, causes exhaustion, and results in confusion. The patient who has this malady can't concentrate enough to do a full day of work or even have a social life. In this case, quality of life definitely suffers, but this isn't considered by much of the medical establishment. In gaslighting those with Long COVID, doctors fail to consider how patients can live with the disease. Instead, they point out that the disease can't possibly exist.

If there is a bright spot in all of this, it's that those with Long COVID have something that those who suffer from chronic fatigue syndrome and fibromyalgia did not. Long COVID patients are pulling together networks of others undergoing the same thing. Online patient communities are bringing Long COVID patients together, as they compare symptoms and commiserate.

Furthermore, because Long COVID seems to impact a large population, those who suffer the symptoms are finding each other and are organizing more quickly to share information and possible lifestyle tools that can help with daily functioning. How this will translate to a higher degree of patient activism and how that activism will continue eroding the doctor-as-gatekeeper and Cartesian dualistic practices remains to be seen. But it's a good example of how patients are taking charge of their health and are seeking solutions that might not be immediately available, or accessible, from traditional medical practices.

The Philosophical and the Physical

There's little doubt that today's clinicians and doctors are facing challenges that their earlier counterparts did not. Granted, the physicians of today have access to all kinds of tools and remedies to help treat once-fatal illnesses and to help ensure longevity. The twenty-first-century physician also must keep up with technological advances, changing market forces, globalization, health care delivery problems, and even the potential of bioterrorism (ABIM Foundation, 2002). Added to that, doctors are asked to handle patients who come from a wide variety of ethnic and cultural backgrounds. This is a fact. In most cases, Western medicine is operating the same way in which it did in the mid-twentieth century. The problem is that this isn't helping today's patients.

Someone who needs medical help these days faces two choices. The person can opt for allopathic, or Western medicine, complete with dualism, gatekeeper mentality, and state-of-the-art technology. This might "cure" what ails, but it doesn't do much else.

That patient could also go the holistic route and find a holistic medical practitioner (Accad, 2016). In this case, the patient might find a more sympathetic ear, but this could also mean a subpar treatment experience. Alternative medical practices can only go so far when it comes to cancer treatments or knee replacements.

As such, neither of these choices is really an ideal solution for the patient. The right solution is to provide the patient with the right tools in order to heal. It means that Western medicine and alternative medicine should find a way to complement one another. In many cases, this is happening, but we're still too far away from providing the patient with healing as opposed to curing.

Western medicine should move away from Cartesian dualism. Instead, today's doctors should incorporate principalism into their methods. This means focusing on patient welfare (serving the patient interest), the principle of patient autonomy (honesty to patients), and the principle of social justice (including fair distribution of healthcare resources).

Furthermore, medicine needs to go back to being an art rather than being stuck solely as a science with a foundation of evidence. Once upon a time, the humanities was essential when it came to the practice of medicine. This has been stripped away, both in the practice and the teaching of medicine. Considering a patient's "lived" experience versus the must-have cause-and-effect scientific requirement of treatment can help the doctor determine the best course of action to relieve a patient's suffering.

Tying philosophy into medical practices means treating the whole patient rather than focusing on the object-body. Medicine with a philosophical bent can relieve the strain on the healthcare system. Instead of sending a patient with CFS, fibromyalgia, or Long COVID to specialists and then through a bewildering series of tests, the doctor should find out how the disease is impacting the patient's quality of life. This means time isn't wasted in trying to "cure" a disease that has no apparent cause. It also means the doctor can avoid medical gaslighting, which can reduce a patient's stress. Certainly, the doctor can treat the symptoms, and should. Tests can be used to confirm a diagnosis (rather than to rule out potential causes). Otherwise, treating patients with a philosophical foundation does a couple of things.

- It reduces the costs and stress of non-essential treatments or drugs; and
- It keeps resources on hand for the patients who truly need them and can benefit from them.

The takeaway of this book is to reintroduce philosophy into the practice of medicine. Doing so requires a wholesale change from the way in which healthcare is delivered and medicine is practiced today.

Philosophy needs to be integrated into the start of medical training. It should be part of the required coursework offered by medical schools, and should be carried over into residency programs. Rather than beating up on interns and residents, and treating these younger doctors with contempt, the entire process of medical training needs to focus on a positive physician-patient partnership. The process also needs to remove the idea that the physician is the all-knowing gatekeeper of medicine while the patient is a reluctant supplicant.

Above all, integration of philosophy into medical treatment enhances respect for patient autonomy. This is stated as a cornerstone of medical practice, but rarely emerges in reality.

The philosophy of social justice in the healthcare system means providing equal healthcare services to all individuals, regardless of their personal characteristics like economic status, age, race, ethnicity, disability, citizenship, or sexual orientation (Habibzadeh, Jasemi, & Hosseinzadegan, 2021). Social justice is also meant to help correct (and hopefully eliminate) inequalities when it comes to maintaining a good level of health care for patients and populations.

Philosophy, Medicine, and the Return to Schiavo

I started this book with an in-depth examination of the Terri Schiavo case. I also pointed out that, had this happened to Terri one hundred years ago, the removal of her PEG and the fight for her life wouldn't have even been an issue. Even though Cartesian dualism was alive and well in the early twentieth century, the means of keeping brain-damaged people alive were non-existent. However, this is what we face with today's medicine. Having the machines to keep people alive even when their brains aren't working highlights the need for more philosophy in medical treatments.

Again, it's not the scope of this paper to determine if Terri's parents or husband were "right" in their struggles. Depending on the school of philosophy that's followed, both sides had their points. We're not here to debate whether Terri's self-determination and autonomy should have been politicized or debated by the courts and then played out in the media, with activists taking on both sides of the issue. It would have been far better to keep the situation a private matter between family members, but it didn't work out that way.

One thing we can take away from this situation is that Terri was regarded more as an "object-body," with the fight between her right to live and her death with dignity. Unfortunately, what the rhetoric, arguing and, yes, the political posturing failed to address was that Terri should have been viewed as a "lived-body" with experiences, wants, hopes, and dreams. Though both her husband and parents indicated that their wishes were to support Terri's best interests, in reality, the interest was more surrounded by what was in the best interests of Michael Schiavo and Mary and Robert Schindler. Michael wanted to end what seemed to be a life not worth living. Mary and Robert simply wanted to keep their little girl alive.

Certainly, there's the argument that Terri should have left an advance directive or living will. Even with that document, philosophical considerations should have been brought into the situation. Issues like quality of life, patient welfare, and patient autonomy could have opened the door to calm, reasonable discussion about how Terri could live her best life. The crime here wasn't that Terri ended her life in a vegetative state, with her PEG removed twice before it came out for good. The crime was that she *was* an object-body. Her autonomy was actively ignored by individuals and politicians who had little medical knowledge but still attempted to play doctor and to believe that they knew Terri's wishes.

As such, evaluating and defining central terms of the medical profession isn't enough to underscore a new approach to medical philosophy. Just evaluating everyone from Plato to Heidegger and beyond can't expand on the practical philosophy of modern medicine. There needs to be a connection between the evaluative process and the practical process. Any kind of philosophy and its ties with medicine should be considered in tandem with the lived human experience, like the culture, society, and history in which patients live.

Thanks to medical technology, the human body can survive all manner of things. However, involving philosophy in the practice of medicine answers the question of existence versus just mere survival. Focusing on philosophy and other branches, like the mind-body connection, physician-patient alliances, and specific quality of life, can bring medical treatment to the humanist side. This, in turn, can benefit patients, doctors, and the overall medical system.

REFERENCES

ABIM Foundation. (2002, February 5). Medical profes-
sionalism in the new millennium: A physician charter.
Annals of Internal Medicine (136), 243–246.

Abimbola, K. (2013, June). Culture and the principles of
biomedical ethics. *Journal of Commercial Biotechnology,*
19(3), 31-39. https://doi.org/10.5912/jcb.598

Accad, M. (2016). How Western medicine lost its soul.
The Linacre Quarterly, 83(2), 144-146.

Au, L., Capotescu, C., Eyal, G., and Finestone, G. (2022).
Long covid and medical gaslighting: Dismissal, delayed
diagnosis, and deferred treatment. *SSM. Qualitative*
Research in Health, 2, 100167. https://doi.org/10.1016/j.
ssmqr.2022.100167

Al-Ghazai, S. K. (2007). *The influence of Islamic philosophy*
and ethics on the development of medicine in the Islamic

civilisation. Retrieved from Foundation for Science Technology and Civilisation: https://www.muslim-heritage.com/uploads/The_Influence_of_Islamic_Philosophy_on_the_Development_of_Medicine.pdf

AMA. (2022, May 15). *What is Long COVID?* Retrieved from American Medical Association: https://www.ama-assn.org/delivering-care/public-health/what-long-covid

American Medical Association. (2023). *Defining basic health care*. Retrieved from AMA Code of Ethics: https://code-medical-ethics.ama-assn.org/ethics-opinions/defining-basic-health-care#:~:text=Health%20care%20is%20a%20fundamental,to%20plan%20for%20our%20lives.

Bhat, A., Parr, T., Ramstead, M., & Friston, K. (2021, April). Immunoceptive inference: Why are psychiatric disorders and immune responses intertwined? *Biology & Philosophy, 36.* https://doi.org/10.1007/s10539-021-09801-6

Bailey, J. E. (2018, December). Socrates' last words to the physical god Asklepios: An ancient call for a healing ethos in civic life. Cureus, 10(2), e3789. https://doi.org/10.7759/cureus.3789

Berlinger, N., & Berlinger, A. (2017, June). Culture and moral distress: What's the connection and why does it matter? *AMA Journal of Ethics, 19*(6), 608-616. https://doi.org/10.1001/journalofethics.2017.19.6.msoc1-1706

Beauchamp, T. L., & Rauprich, O. (2016). Principalism. In *Encyclopedia of Global Bioethics* (pp. 2282-2293). Cham, Switzerland: Springer Chamb.

Bishop, J. P. (2009). Biopolitics, Terri Schiavo and the sovereign subject of death. *Journal of Medicine and Philosophy, 33*, 538-557. https://doi.org/10.1093/jmp/jhn029

Blease, C., Carel, H., & Geraghty, K. (2017). Epistemic injustice in healthcare encounters: evidence from chronic fatigue syndrome. *Journal of Medical Ethics, 43*, 549-557. doi:10.1136/medethics-2016-103691

Boss, J. (1978). The medical philosophy of Francis Bacon (1561-1626). *Medical Hypotheses, 4*(3), 208-220. https://doi.org/10.1016/0306-9877(78)90003-8

Boudreau, R. (2018). The relevance of existential philosophy in medicine. *Journal of Clinical Research & Bioethics, 9*(3). https://doi.org/10.4172/2155-9627.1000326

Boylan, M. (n.d.). *Hippocrates* (c. 450–380 BCE). Retrieved from Internet Encyclopedia of Philosophy: https://iep. utm.edu/hippocra/

Bradley, K. L., Goetz, T., & Viswanathan, S. (2018, November–December). Toward a contemporary definition of health. *Military Medicine, 183*(3), 204-207. https://doi.org/10.1093/milmed/usy213

Brazier, Y. (2018, November 16). *What was ancient Egyptian medicine like?* Retrieved from Medical News Today: https://www.medicalnewstoday.com/articles/323633

Breed, A. G., & Crenson, M. (2006, March 26). *What do the Schiavo videotapes really show?* Retrieved from NBC News: https://www.nbcnews.com/id/wbna7303236

Britannica, T. Editors of Encyclopedia (2023, May 15). *Philosophy.* Retrieved from Encyclopedia Britannica. https://www.britannica.com/topic/philosophy

Brower, V. (2006). Mind–body research moves towards the mainstream. *EMBO Reports, 7*(4). https://doi.org/10.1038/sj.embor.7400671

Bottalico, L., Charitos, I. A., Kolveris, N., D'Agostino, D., Topi, S., Ballini, A., & Santacroce, L. (2019). Philosophy and Hippocratic Ethic in Ancient Greek Society: Evolution of Hospital—Sanctuaries. Open Access: *Macedonian Journal of Medical Sciences, 7*(19), 3353–3357. https://doi.org/10.3889/oamjms.2019.474

Chalasani, R. (2016, March 31). *A look back: The Terri Schiavo case.* Retrieved from CBS News: https://www.cbsnews.com/pictures/look-back-in-history-terri-schiavo-death/

Chan, E., Ahmed, T., Wang, M., & Chan, J. (1994). History of medicine and nephrology in Asia. *American Journal of Nephrology, 14*, 295-301.

Charatan, F. (2005, March). President Bush and Congress intervene in "right to die" case. *BMJ, 330*(7493), 687. https://doi.org/10.1136/bmj.330.7493.687-a

Cleveland Clinic. (2023). *Hypoxemia.* Retrieved from Cleveland Clinic: https://my.clevelandclinic.org/health/diseases/17727-hypoxemia

Collyer, F. M., Willis, K. F., & Lewis, S. (2017, August). Gatekeepers in the healthcare sector: Knowledge and Bourdieu's concept of field. *Social Science & Medicine, 186*, 96-103. https://doi.org/10.1016/j.socscimed.2017.06.004

Conrad, L. I., Neve, M., Nutton, V., Porter, R., & Wear, A. (1995). *The Western Medical Tradition: 800 BC to AD 1800 (1ˢᵗ Edition)*. New York, NY: Cambridge University Press.

Conti, A. A. (2012). Historical evolution of the concept of health in Western medicine. *Acta Biomed, 89*(3), 352-354. https://doi.org/10.23750/abm.v89i3.6739

Dictionary.com. (2023). *Healthcare*. Retrieved from Dictionary.com: https://www.dictionary.com/browse/healthcare#:~:text=noun%20Also%20health%20care%20.,healthcare%20workers%3B%20a%20healthcare%20center.

Doolittle, B. R. (2021, April). The philosopher-priest-scientist and the new age of medicine. *The American Journal of Medicine, 134*(4), 425-426. https://doi.org/10.1016/j.amjmed.2020.12.006

Edwards, S. A. (2012, March 1). *Paracelsus, the man who brought chemistry to medicine*. Retrieved from American Association for the Advancement of Science: https://www.aaas.org/paracelsus-man-who-brought-chemistry-medicine

Elkington, J. (1966, March). Medicine and the quality of life. *Annals of Internal Medicine, 64*, 711-714.

Fenigsen, R. (2011). Other people's lives: reflection on medicine, ethics and euthanasia, part two: medicine versus euthanasia. *Issues in Law & Medicine, 26*(3), 239-279.

Ferngren, G. B. (2009). *Medicine and Health Care in Early Christianity.* Baltimore, MD: Johns Hopkins University Press.

Frey, E. (1985). The earliest medical texts. *Clio Medica, 20*(1-4), 79-90.

Friedland, G. (2009, May). Discovery of the function of the heart and circulation of the blood. *Cardiovascular Journal of Africa,* 20(3), 160.

Freudenthal, R. (2021, December 3). *The medical objectification of the human person.* Retrieved from The Brownstone Institute: https://brownstone.org/articles/the-medical-objectification-of-the-human-person/

Giglioni, G. (2012). *Francis Bacon.* Retrieved from Stanford Encyclopedia of Philosophy: https://plato.stanford.edu/entries/francis-bacon/

Habibzadeh, H., Jasemi, M., & Hosseinzadegan, F. (2021). Social justice in health system a neglected component of academic nursing education: A qualitative study. *BMC Nursing, 20,* 16. https://doi.org/10.1186/ s12912-021-00534-1

Hajar, R. (2015). History of medicine timeline. *Heart Views, 16*(1), 43–45. https://doi.org/10.4103/1995-705x.153008

Haraldstad, K., Wahl, A., Andenaes, R., Andersen, J., Andersen, M., Beisland, E., Helseth, S. (2019, June). A systematic review of quality of life research in medicine and health sciences. *Quality of Life Research, 28,* 2641–2650.

Haque, O. S., & Waytz, A. (2012). Dehumanization in medicine: causes, solutions, and functions. *Perspectives on Psychological Science, 7*(2), 176–187. https://doi.org/1 0.1016/10.1177/1/45691611429706

Hatfield, G. (2014). *Rene Descartes.* Retrieved from Stanford Encyclopedia of Philosophy: https://plato.stanford.edu/ entries/descartes/

Hook, C., & Mueller, P. (2005, November). The Terri Schiavo saga: The making of a tragedy and lessons learned. *Mayo Clinical Proceedings, 80*(11), 1449–1460.

Huffman, C. (2021, Summer). *Alcmaeon.* Retrieved from The Standard Encyclopedia of Philosophy: https://plato.stanford.edu/archives/sum2021/entries/alcmaeon/

Johns Hopkins Medicine. (2023). *Stomach and duodenal ulcers (peptic ulcers).* Retrieved from Johns Hopkins Medicine: https://www.hopkinsmedicine.org/health/conditions-and-diseases/stomach-and-duodenal-ulcers-peptic-ulcers

Karff, S. E. (2009, October). Recognizing the mind/body/spirit connection in medical care. *American Medical Association Journal of Ethics, 11*(10), 788-792.

Keller, S. (2009, January). Welfarism. Philosophy *Compas, 4*(1), 82-95. https://doi.org/10.1111/j.1747-9991.2008.00196.x

King, L. S. (1954, January). Plato's concepts of medicine. *Journal of the History of Medicine and Allied Sciences, 9*(1), 38-48.

Kirkengen, A., Ekeland, T.-J., Getz, L., Hetlevik, I., Schei, E., Ulvestad, E., & Vetlesen, A. J. (2016). Medicine's perception of reality -- a split picture: Critical reflections on apparent anomalies within the biomedical theory of science. *Journal of Evaluation in*

Clinical Practice, 22, 496-501. https://doi.org/10.1111/ jep.12369

Kitzinger, J., & Kitzinger, C. (2013, September). The "window of opportunity" for death after severe brain injury: family experiences. *Sociology of Health & Illness, 35*(7), 1095-1112. https://doi.org/10.1111/1467-9566.12020

Koch, T. (2005, July). The challenge of Terri Schiavo: Lessons for bioethics. *Journal of Medical Ethics, 31*(7), 376-378. https://doi.org/10.1136%2Fjme.2005.012419

Kuhse, H., & Singer, P. (1989). The quality/quantity-of-life distinction and its moral importance for nurses. *International Journal of Nursing Studies, 26*(3), 203-212. https://doi.org/10.1016/0020-7489(89)90001-1

Majeed, A. (2005, December). How Islam changed medicine. *BMJ, 331*(7531), 1486-1487. https://doi.org/10.1136/ bmj.331.7531.1486

Mantri, S. (2008, March). History of medicine: Holistic medicine and the western medical tradition. *American Medical Association Journal of Ethics, 10*(3), 177-180. https:// doi.org/10.1001/virtualmentor.2008.10.3.mhst1-0803

Marcum, J. A. (n.d.). *Philosophy of medicine*. Retrieved from Internet Encyclopedia of Philosophy: https://iep. utm.edu/medicine/

Mark, J. J. (2020, October 16). *Philosophy*. Retrieved from World History Encyclopedia: https://www.worldhistory.org/philosophy/

Masic, I., Miokovic, M., & Muhamedagic, B. (2008). Evidence-based medicine -- new approaches and challenges. *Acta Informatica Medica, 16*(4), 219-225. https://doi.org/10.5455/aim.2008.16.219-225

Mechanic D. (2001). The managed care backlash: perceptions and rhetoric in health care policy and the potential for health care reform. *The Milbank Quarterly, 79*(1), 35–VI. https://doi.org/10.1111/1468-0009.00195

Metwaly, A. M., Ghoneim, M. M., Eissa, I. H., Elsehemy, I. A., Mostafa, A. E., Hegazy, M. M., Afifi, W. M., & Dou, D. (2021). Traditional ancient Egyptian medicine: A review. *Saudi Journal of Biological Sciences, 28*(10), 5823–5832. https://doi.org/10.1016/j.sjbs.2021.06.044

Moes M. (2001). Plato's conception of the relations between moral philosophy and medicine. *Perspectives in Biology and Medicine, 44*(3), 353–367. <u>https://doi.</u> <u>org/10.1353/pbm.2001.0055</u>

Moore, A. (2013). *Hedonism.* Retrieved from Stanford Encyclopedia of Philosophy: <u>https://plato.stanford.</u> <u>edu/entries/hedonism/</u>

Musschenga, A. W. (1997, February). The relation between concepts of quality-of-life, health and happiness. *The Journal of Medicine and Philosophy: A Forum for Bioethics and Philosophy of Medicine, 22*(1), 11-28. https://doi.org/10.1093/jmp/22.1.11

NIH. (2023). *Fibromyalgia.* Retrieved from National Institute of Arthritis and Musculoskeletal and Skin Diseases: https://www.niams.nih.gov/health-topics/fibromyalgia#:~:text=Fibromyalgia%20is%20a%20chronic%20 (long,a%20heightened%20sensitivity%20to%20pain.

NLM. (2012, February 7). *Greek Medicine.* Retrieved from National Library of Medicine, History of Medicine Division, National Institutes of Health: <u>https://www.</u> <u>nlm.nih.gov/hmd/greek/greek_oath.html</u>

Nantais, D., & Kuczewksi, M. (2004). Quality of life: The contested rhetoric of resource allocation and end-of-life decision making. *Journal of Medicine and Philosophy, 29*(6), 651–664.

National Geographic. (2020). *Taoism.* Retrieved from National Geographic: https://education.nationalgeo-graphic.org/resource/taoism

Nutton, V. (2023, February). *Galen.* Retrieved from Britannica: https://www.britannica.com/biography/Galen

Pennacchini, M., Bertolaso, M., Elvira, M., & DeMarinis, M. (2011). A brief history of the Quality of Life: Its use in medicine and in philosophy. *La Clinica Terapeutica, 162*(3), e99–e103.

Putt, S. S., Wijeakumar, S., Franciscus, R. G., & Spencer, J. P. (2017). The functional brain networks that underlie Early Stone Age tool manufacture. *Nature Human Behaviour, 1*(0102). https://doi.org/10.1038/s41562-017-0102

Rajshekhar, C., El-Jawahri, A., Litzow, M. R., Syrjala, K. L., Parnes, A. D., & Hashmi, S. (2017). A systematic review of religious beliefs about major end-of-life issues in the five major world religions. *Palliative Support Care, 15*(5), 609–622. https://doi.org/10.1017/S1478951516001061

Rankin, L. (2011, October 11). The difference between healing and curing. Retrieved from Psychology Today: https://www.psychologytoday.com/us/blog/owning-pink/201110/the-difference-between-healing-and-curing

Raphals, L. (2020, Winter). *Chinese philosophy and Chinese medicine.* Retrieved from The Stanford Encyclopedia of Philosophy: https://plato.stanford.edu/archives/win2020/entries/chinese-phil-medicine/

Reiss, J. (2016, June 6). *Philosophy of medicine.* Retrieved from Stanford Encyclopedia of Philosophy: https://plato.stanford.edu/entries/medicine/

Risse, G. (1986, May). Imhotep and medicine -- a reevaluation. Western Journal of Medicine, 144(5), 622-624.

Rotaru, T.-Ş., Popa, T., & Cuza, A. I. (2020, June). How can Plato be relevant for contemporary medicine? *Journal of Intercultural Management and Ethics* (2), 59-66. https://doi.org/10.35478/jime.2020.2.07

Sallam, H. (2012). The ancient Alexandria school of medicine. Gynecologie, Obstetrique & Fertilite, 30(1), 3-10. https://doi.org/10.1016/s1297-9589(01)00254-5

Sallam H. N. (2010). Aristotle, godfather of evidence-based medicine. *Facts, Views & Vision in ObGyn, 2*(1), 11–19.

Samuel, A., & Bowman, A. K. (n.d.). Macedonian and Ptolemaic Egypt (332-30 BCE). Retrieved from Britannica: https://www.britannica.com/place/ancient-Egypt/Government-and-conditions-under-the-Ptolemies

Sartorius, N. (2006, August). The meanings of health and its promotion. *Croatian Medical Journal, 47*(4), 6620664.

Schramme, T. (2015). Philosophy of Medicine and Bioethics. In T. Schramme, & S. Edwards (Eds.), *Handbook of the Philosophy of Medicine* (pp. 3-15). Dordrecht, United Kingdom: Springer Science + Business Media.

Sebring, J. C. (2021, November). Towards a sociological understanding of medical gaslighting in western health care. *Sociology of Health & Illness, 43*(9), 1951-1964. https://doi.org/10.1111/1467-9566.13367

Selig, M. (2021, December 1). *Does it matter if you dislike your doctor?* Retrieved from Psychology Today: https://www.psychologytoday.com/us/blog/changepower/202112/does-it-matter-if-you-dislike-your-doctor

Sigerist, H. E. (2018). *Civilization and Disease*. Ithaca, New York: Cornell University Press.

Sinnott-Armstrong, W. (2019, January). *Consequentialism*. (2019, Editor) Retrieved from Stanford Encyclopedia of Philosophy: https://plato.stanford.edu/entries/consequentialism/

Stempsey, W. E. (2008, Summer). Philosophy of medicine is what philosophers of medicine do. *Perspectives in Biology and Medicine, 51*(3), 379-391.

Stoppler, M. C. (2021, March 29). *Medical definition of quality of life*. Retrieved from MedicineNet: https://www.medicinenet.com/quality_of_life/definition.htm

Tai, D., Shah, A., Doubeni, C., Sia, I., & Wieland, M. (2021, February). The disproportionate impact of COVID-19 on racial and ethnic minorities in the United States. *Clinical Infectious Diseases, 72*(4), 703-706. https://doi.org/10.1093/cid/ciaa815

Taylor, S. C. (n.d.). *Health care ethics*. Retrieved from Internet Encyclopedia of Philosophy: https://iep.utm.edu/h-c-ethi/

ten Have, H., & Gordijn, B. (2019). Education and the soul of medicine. *Medicine, Health Care and Philosophy* (22), 165-166. https://doi.org/10.1007/s11019-019-09894-7

Thoma, A., & Eaves, F. F. (2015, November-December). A brief history of evidence-based medicine (EBM) and the contributions of Dr. David Sackett. *Aesthetic Surgery Journal, 35*(8), NP261-NP263. https://doi.org/10.1093/asj/sjv130

Timmermans, S., & Almeling, R. (2009, August). Objectification, standardization and commoditization in health care: A conceptual readjustment. *Social Science & Medicine, 69*, 21-27. https://doi.org/10.1016/j.socscimed.2009.04.020

Tosam, Mbih Jerome. 2014. "The Role of Philosophy in Modern Medicine." *Open Journal of Philosophy* 4, no. 1 (February): 75–84. http://dx.doi.org/10.4236/ojpp.2014.41011.

Tsiompanou, E., & Marketos, S. G. (2013, July). Hippocrates: Timeless still. *Journal of the Royal Society of Medicine, 106*(7), 288-292.

US National Library of Medicine. (2000). *Classics of traditional Chinese medicine.* Retrieved from History

of Medicine: https://www.nlm.nih.gov/exhibition/
chinesemedicine/emperors.html#:~:text=Shen%20
Nung%20%E7%A5%9E%E8%BE%B2%20is%20
venerated,introduced%twentiethe%20technique%20
of%20acupuncture.

Vitetta, L., Anton, B., Cortizo, F., & Sali, A. (2005, December). Mind-body medicine: Stress and its impact on overall health and longevity. *Annals of the New York Academy of Sciences, 1057*(1), 492-505. https://doi.org/10.1111/j.1749-6632.2005.tb06153.x

Taylor, S. C. (n.d.). *Health care ethics*. Retrieved from Internet Encyclopedia of Philosophy: https://iep.utm.edu/h-c-ethi/

WHO. (2022). *WHO constitution*. Retrieved from World Health Organization: https://www.who.int/about/governance/constitution

WHOQOL Group. (1995, November). The World Health organization quality of life assessment (WHOQOL): Position paper from the World Health Organization. *Social Science & Medicine, 41*(10), 1403-1409. https://doi.org/10.1016/0277-9536(95)00112-K

West, J. B. (2014, July). Galen and the beginnings of Western physiology. *American Journal of Physiology, 307*(2), 121-128. https://doi.org/10.1152/ajplung.00123.2014

Wheeler, M. (2011, October 12). *Martin Heidegger.* Retrieved from Stanford Encyclopedia of Philosophy: https://plato.stanford.edu/entries/heidegger/

Wolfson, J. (2006, March). The basis for decisions to end life. The Schiavo dilemma: An essay by the Special Guardian Ad Litem. *Clinical Interventions in Aging, 1*(1), 3-6. https://doi.org/10.2147/ciia.2006.1.1.3

Wulff, H. (1992). Philosophy of medicine -- from a medical perspective. *Theoretical Medicine and Bioethics, 13,* 79-85.

Zahir, I. I. (2016, September). Hippocrates: Philosophy and medicine. European Scientific Journal, 12(26), 199-210. https://doi.org/10.19044/esj.2016.v12n26p199

Zapata, J. A., & Moriates, C. (2015, November). The high-value care considerations of inpatient versus out-patient testing. *American Medical Association Journal of Ethics, 17*(1), 1022-1027.

INDEX

cultural health capital, 105
culture
    defined, 137–138
    and health care, 137–141
curing, healing as compared to,
    48–49, 64
Curzan, Nancy, xvi–xvii

D
Daoism (Taoism), 11, 12, 13
death with dignity, xii–xx, 109,
    117, 138, 177
dehumanization/depersonaliza-
    tion, of Western medicine,
    44, 52, 62, 98, 99, 100,
    101, 103
dementia, 120–121
deontology, 132–133
Descartes, Rene, 53–54, 56
diet, emphasis on in Greek medi-
    cine, 27
discours de La Methode (Descartes),
    53–54
disease, according to
    Hippocrates, 28
doctors. *See also* physicians
    as all knowing, 95, 175.
        See also gatekeeper
        mentality
    "major deity," as meaning of
        MD, 102
    as suffering from mechanized
        focus of today's medi-
        cine, 101
do-not-resuscitate orders, 125

dry, as one of four primary qual-
    ities, 31
dying, medical aid in, 118

E
Ebers Medical Papyrus, 4
EBM (evidence-based medicine)
    criticism of, 74–75
    as fitting under utilitarian
        philosophy, 131
    versus PCM, 155–157
    rise and practice of, 73–75, 79
Edwin Smith Surgical Papyrus, 4
efficiency
    as one of Aristotle's four
        causal categories, 153
    as one of Bacon's two causal
        categories, 154
Egypt, ancient, role of in medi-
    cine, 3–9
Elkington, J. R., 111
The Epic of Gilgamesh, 2
epistemology, 152–153
Erasistratus, 9
ethics, defined, 127–130
euthanasia, 118–121
evidence-based medicine (EBM)
    criticism of, 74–75
    as fitting under utilitarian
        philosophy, 131
    versus PCM, 155–157
    rise and practice of, 73–75, 79
Eyal, G., 170–171

F
"female issues," use of phrase, 72

201

Fenigsen, Richard, 118–119
fibromyalgia, 70–71, 72
final cause, as one of Aristotle's
    four causal categories, 153
Finestone, G., 170–171
Florida, Terri's Law, xv, xvii,
    xviii–xix
formal, as one of Aristotle's four
    causal categories, 153
Foucault, Michel, xvii
Freudenthal, Robert, 45
Frist, Bill, xv, 107

G
Galen of Pergamum, 9, 30–36,
    37, 42
gatekeeper mentality, of Western
    medicine, 105, 162, 172,
    173, 175
Ge Hong, 12
gender bias, in health care, 71–72
glioblastoma multiforme (GBM),
    131–133
Greece, ancient
    health care decision-making
        in, 127
    role of in medicine, 13–30
    role of in philosophy, 2

H
Han Dynasty (China), 10
Harvey, William, 33, 38, 42–43
Hawking, Stephen, 91, 92
healing
    as compared to curing, 48–
        49, 64

and mental/emotional con-
    nection, 62–66
mind-body for, 155–157
health
    defined, 89–91, 93–94
    quality of life (QOL) versus,
        124–125
health care, defined, 92
health care delivery/health care
    system
    culture and, 137–141
    current one as far from sus-
        tainable, 104
    limitations of current
        modes, 102
    managed care in, 87, 88
    minority groups as having
        less access to, 138
    overview, 75–79
health maintenance organizations
    (HMOs), 87
health-related quality of life
    (HRQOL), 112, 114
Hearst Medical Papyrus, 4
hedonism, and QOL debate,
    117–118
Heidegger, Martin, 165–166
Herophlus, 9
Hesiod, 15
Hippocrates of Cos, 4, 8, 13,
    21–30, 36
Hippocratic Corpus, 21, 25–30, 142
Hippocratic Oath, 22, 24–25
HMOs (health maintenance or-
    ganizations), 87
holism, 147–149

mind-body connection, ix, xix, 40, 62, 68, 144, 155–157, 165, 166–167, 178

mind-body separation, 54

mind-body-soul connection, 33, 34, 35, 38, 73, 101, 126

mind-body-soul separation, 43, 57–62, 142

mindfulness, 66, 72, 82, 148

morbidity and mortality conferences, 101

Moriates, C., 83–85, 88–89

MRSA (methicillin-resistant Staphylococcus aureus), 85

N

National Institutes of Health, Office of Alternative Medicine, 162

nonmaleficence, 104, 134, 136

nurses, as suffering from mechanized focus of today's medicine, 101

O

object-bodies, patients as, 52, 62, 80–81, 104, 133, 162, 168, 174, 177, 178

ocular migraine, 79

Office of Alternative Medicine (NIH), 162

office-centered care, of Western medicine, 78

ontological reductionism, 145–147, 149

ontology, 151–152

opium, tincture, origins of, 38

Opus Paramirum (Paracelsus), 39

Ornish, Dean, 159

P

pain. *See also* fibromyalgia; migraines

    as all in the patient's mind, 68–69

    causes of, 67–68

    chronic pain, 69

    defined, 67

    treating of as holistic issue, 72–73

papyri, 3–4, 6–7

Paracelsus, 38–42, 54

patient autonomy, xviii, xix, 103, 109, 121, 122, 128, 133–134, 135, 136, 137, 161, 173, 175, 176, 177–178

patient care, depersonalization of. *See* dehumanization/depersonalization, of Western medicine

patient mix-ups, 101

patients

    as cost generators, 93

    depersonalization and dehumanization of, 44, 52, 62, 98, 100, 101, 103

    as left out of diagnosis and treatment, 83

    as lived-bodies, 81–82, 104, 133, 160, 174, 177

"window of opportunity,"
  with brain injuries/brain
  death, 109
"window shade theory," 40
Wolfson, Jay, 108
World Health Organization
    (WHO)
  on health, 90
  on quality of life (QOL), 112
Wuff, Henrick, 143–144

Y

yellow bile, as one of four humors, 26, 27
yin and yang, 13

Z

Zapata, J. A., 83–85, 88–89
Zhou Dynasty (China), 10

www.ingramcontent.com/pod-product-compliance
Lightning Source LLC
Chambersburg PA
CBHW021358210526
45463CB00001B/149